# REFLECTIONS OF CARE

# A CENTURY OF NURSING IN CAPE BRETON

Cape Breton Retired Nurses Interest Group

Edited by

Donna Anderson Currie
Tom Ayers

Chief Advisor

Robert Morgan

Cape Breton University Press Inc.

Sydney, Nova Scotia

Cape Breton University Press recognizes the support of the Province of Nova Scotia, through the Department of Tourism, Culture and Heritage. We are pleased to work in partnership with the Culture Division to develop and promote our cultural resources for Nova Scotians.

NOVA SCOTIA
Tourism, Culture and Heritage

Cover Design: Cathy MacLean, Pleasant Bay, NS
Layout: Mike Hunter, Louisbourg, NS
Printing by Marquis Book Publishing, Cap Ste Ignace

**Library and Archives Canada Cataloguing in Publication**

Reflections of care : a century of nursing in Cape Breton / edited by Donna Anderson Currie, Tom Ayers, Robert Morgan.
Includes index.

ISBN 1-897009-16-X
    1. Nursing--Nova Scotia--Cape Breton Island--History. 2. Nursing--Study and teaching--Nova Scotia--Cape Breton Island--History.
I. Currie, Donna Anderson II. Ayers, Tom, 1962- III. Morgan, Robert J.
RT6.N6R43 2006      610.73'097169      C2006-905883-0

Cape Breton University Press
PO Box 5300
Sydney, NS  B1P 6L2
Canada

To those who went before:

It is on your shoulders that we stand

It is in your footsteps that we tread.

Anon.

REFLECTIONS OF CARE

A CENTURY OF NURSING IN CAPE BRETON

Cape Breton Retired Nurses Interest Group

Contents

The Nightingale Pledge 7

Preface 9

Foreword 11

Nursing Issues 1930–2000 13

Nursing Schools of Cape Breton and Beyond
and Featured Graduates 19

Graduate Reflections and Local Highlights 23

Glace Bay 25
New Waterford 57
Sydney 73
North Sydney / Sydney Mines 113
Victoria County 143
Inverness County 155
Richmond County 177

Index 182

Sponsors 183

# NIGHTINGALE PLEDGE

I solemnly pledge myself before God and in the presence
of this assembly:

To pass my life in purity and to practise my profession faithfully.

I will abstain from whatever is deleterious and mischievous, and
will not take or knowingly administer any harmful drug.

I will do all in my power to elevate the standard of my profession,
and will hold in confidence all personal matters committed to
my keeping and all family affairs coming to my knowledge in the
practise of my profession.

With loyalty will I endeavour to aid the physician in his work and
devote myself to the welfare of those committed to my care.

The Nightingale pledge is an oath frequently taken by nurses at
capping ceremonies or upon graduation from a school of nursing.
It was written in 1895 by a committee of which Mrs. Lystra E. Green
was chair and was first administered to the 1895 graduating class of
the Farrand Training School, Harper Hospital, Detroit, Michigan.

# PREFACE

By Donna Anderson Currie, editor

During the span of a year, I had the pleasure of reading the career memories of more than sixty nurses from Cape Breton. The first nurse featured graduated in 1916. A few began their careers in the 1930s and 1940s, while many started out in the 1950s and 60s. There were also a couple of contributions from nurses who graduated in the 1970s and as late as 1980. Obviously the stories come from different eras; what struck me most as I read and edited were not the differences, but the similarities.

As so many of those interviewed noted, nursing is more than a career. For many it is a way of life that doesn't end with retirement. Readers will recognize other common experiences in the interviews, beginning with the memory of the limited career choices facing women upon high school graduation until quite recently. Teacher, nurse or secretary—what would it be? The challenges and stereotypes facing male nurses are also remembered.

The camaraderie and bonds established during training were emphasized. Nurses recalled their strict, hands-on education. They entered the workplace with the confidence of those who were well prepared. Pregnant nurses and working mothers often were not welcome in hospitals until the 1960s, but the profession offered flexible and portable job opportunities. Many single parents used their nursing careers to support families.

The changing role of nurses was a hot topic among interviewed retirees. While many are very comfortable with today's nursing education, there is some concern that degree programs don't graduate enough nurses who are ready for general duty. Changes to nurses' uniforms emerged as a minor bone of contention as well. There is some suggestion among contributors that nurses need to be easily identified by their patients and that current dress codes can create confusion.

Retirees told us that nursing is a physically and mentally demanding profession. Many retired early due to injury, burnout and/or the pressures of staff shortages and cutbacks, important issues for the future of health care.

Editing these nursing memories has led me to reflect on the nurses in my own life and particularly those most important to me: my aunts Allie Taylor and Margie Morrissey. They have always exemplified the nursing qualities reflected in these interviews— caring, compassionate and dedicated. I dedicate my work on this project to them.

D.A.C.
North Sydney

Publisher's note: The reflections included in this collection are written from interview transcriptions and every effort has been made to ensure that nothing was lost as the spoken word was made into the written word. Content, tense, grammar and syntax are preserved as much as possible in the spirit of the telling.

The reflections are organized by the communities with which the subjects are most often identified.

The opinions expressed are those of the featured graduates themselves.

# FOREWORD

## CAPE BRETON RETIRED NURSES INTEREST GROUP

The idea for this book originated from a chance meeting about seven years ago at the Cape Breton Regional Hospital between Frances Ellison, Carolyn Richards and myself. The three of us had a cumulative total of more than 100 years of nursing experience, much of it in Cape Breton. We were in a reflective mood, pondering the history of the noble profession of nursing on our beautiful island; our conversation focused on the impressive setting of the new hospital. Soon our thoughts led to the need to capture the stories and culture of the nurses who served the three original hospitals that had amalgamated to create the new facility.

In 2002, some members of the recently established Cape Breton Retired Nurses Interest Group Society were searching for a project. Mildred Kettlewell, Marilyn Morrison Foley, Marion Hopkins, Ethel Cluett, Tula Gouthro and I returned to the original idea of compiling nursing history narratives from the previous hospitals and soon the concept grew. We developed the notion of accumulating oral histories from retired nurses regarding their education and career experiences. This was a novel and innovative project. There was no documentation available on Cape Breton nurses who had graduated from local hospital nursing schools. Other nurses had been educated off the island, some in the traditional hospital setting, others from university programs.

This book seeks to remedy that omission and highlight the various nursing programs offered in Cape Breton from 1900–2000, to honour, celebrate and document our rich nursing experiences.

As our project idea developed, the federal government was funding a five-year social research project in Cape Breton known as the Community Employment Innovation Project (CEIP). Our committee received money to hire two people to conduct interviews with Cape Breton nurses over a period of two years. Rose Gillis and Laurie Marazek began this Herculean task in 2003, conducting research at the Beaton Institute. Local author and historian Dr. Robert Morgan, former director of the Beaton Institute, Cape Breton University, agreed to join our project as an advisor. In 2004, through a Human Resources and Skills Development Canada grant, journalism student Laura MacInnis was hired and was invaluable in completing the final interviews.

Special mention must be given to Rose Gillis who organized the interviews and the office on Lingan Road. We would also like to thank Lem Skeete for the provision of free office space at the United Mission and the CEIP staff for their help and support. The project was approved thanks to the District Innovation Project Association Board.

Interviewees were recruited through society meetings, media coverage and the Council of the College of Registered Nurses of Nova Scotia College newsletter. Dr. Morgan assisted in developing questions designed to create a consistent format. Each nurse's story was recorded during two-hour individual interviews held in communities across Cape Breton in 2003 and 2004. Nurses not available for in-person interviews responded to the questions by mail. The conversations were then transcribed and reviewed by the committee and by Dr. Morgan. We selected sixty-seven of those that we felt best reflected the spirit of the project. Those chosen were sent to writer Donna Anderson Currie for editing. All nurses later reviewed the edited interviews for accuracy.

The interviews were then further edited by Tom Ayers for readability and to follow suggestions of the publisher. Every effort was made to maintain the flavour and intent of the interviews.

We owe an immense debt of gratitude to those nurses who generously gave of their time to participate in this exciting endeavour. Thank you to the many people who supported us throughout this entire project and special thanks to Kay Stephenson, Dr. Simone Roach, Claire Currie and Charmaine MacPherson (PhD Nusing candidate).

Clotilda Yakimchuk, Chairperson

# NURSING ISSUES
## 1900–2000

In the early 1900s, Canadian nursing schools were identified with hospital ownership and administration. These in-house diploma programs and a few university degree programs provided excellent resources for service and education.

From the 1930s onward, evolving world events radically changed the manner in which nurses trained and practised. Major influences in the 1930s and 1940s included military, religious and family and social values and cultural change.

### THE IMPACT OF WAR

The impact of the two world wars brought nurses near the front lines of combat in Europe. War accelerated adjustments in the delivery of care to the wounded and promoted change in health care service at home, generating a need for creative approaches in the care of the sick and the preparation of caregivers.

Jewish- and Christian-sponsored health care facilities throughout Canada shaped the values by which services were provided. These same values shaped family life in rural and urban communities. Student nurses of the time often came from large families and entered nursing school already groomed by emphasis on responsibility, hard work, compassion for the sick and concern for one's neighbour. The transition to nursing school discipline and residence was natural for most students. Those who chose nursing in the 1930s and 1940s were motivated by the influence of Florence Nightingale and nurtured by the religious influence of their particular faith.

This time period was not without its growing pains and struggles. The tension between service demands and the need for upgrading in both educational environments and in the nursing schools continued throughout this period. Those involved in both service and education knew too well the tension between providing the best service to patients while maintaining the high educational and practice standards demanded of nursing schools.

The demobilization of servicemen following World War II resulted in a major population increase and a resulting increase in the demand for prenatal care. Nurses who served in the war brought home acquired concepts of nursing care for mass casualties. Their knowledge was invaluable to hospitals preparing to deal with the aftermath of nuclear explosions during the height of the Cold War. These nurses became involved in many facets of disaster planning.

Coronary care and intensive care units grew with a resulting increase in specialty training. Managers and administrators required advanced preparation and master's- and doctoral-level programs increased. The national Medicare program brought massive changes in nurse-to-patient ratios, delivery of service and financial accountability. The general public joined the governing councils of professional nursing organizations and a new era of review and restructuring began. The introduction and development of nursing research utilization generated a focus on nursing practice based on scientific studies.

## A NEW ERA

Prior to the 1950s, psychiatric care was largely custodial. In the 1960s and 1970s , although electro-convulsive therapy and hydrotherapy were used, new approaches such as psychotropic drugs, psychotherapy and insulin therapy became treatments of choice. The philosophy of care changed to include group homes, development of outpatient clinics, shorter hospital stays and discharge planning.

Working conditions for nurses became a key issue in the 1960s in areas of salary, benefits, work scheduling and lifestyle. It was during these times that collective bargaining began for nursing. In 1975, the first provincial nurses' strike took place. In Cape

Breton, the strike was led by the late Theresa Murphy of St. Rita Hospital, union president. This was a significant time for nursing. A profession that had been primarily female was making a strong stand for equity, quality of work life and better pay. Nurses were developing a voice, a struggle that continues. Nursing standards of practice became the focus of professional nursing associations, resulting in changes to the required basic competencies for the registered nurse. More definitive job descriptions were introduced and performance appraisals defined accountability.

During the 1970s and 1980s, Cape Breton was well represented at the Registered Nurses Association of Nova Scotia, now known as the College of Registered Nurses of Nova Scotia. Gladys Smith was president from 1976 to 1978 and Clotilda Yakimchuk was in the role from 1986 to 1988. In the 1980s, the RNANS expanded to include representatives from the general public. Communications Professor Dr. Mary Lynch of the University College of Cape Breton (now Cape Breton University) joined the board of directors. In 1984, the Cape Breton branch of RNANS won the Branch of the Year Award after developing a Sydney evening clinic for seniors offering blood pressure and glucose testing, weight assessments and medication reviews. Local nurses were already aware of the importance of health promotion and education.

Continuous quality improvement programs were adapted for health care organizations. New technology began to have an impact on nursing. Disposable items such as needles, syringes, tubing, catheters and gloves were introduced. Workload measurement systems were introduced. This conflicted with the nursing role, failing to measure the caring so important to nursing. A provincial home care program reduced hospital stays and increased the need for collaboration between all members of the health care team.

New nursing roles were developed including clinical nurse practitioners, patient educators, patient advocates and in-service, diabetes and education coordinators. The multi-disciplinary approach to care was introduced and mission statements describing visions and values of care were developed. Nursing care plans based on nursing diagnosis with identified patient outcomes became common practice.

## INCREASING EDUCATION REQUIREMENTS

As in-service coordinators were hired at hospital sites in Cape Breton, the Cape Breton Continuing Education Committee was formed to ensure quality staff education. Founding members were Mildred Kettlewell of the Northside General Hospital, Yvonne Boone at the Sydney City Hospital, Jean Rose at St. Rita Hospital, Clotilda Yakimchuk at Cape Breton Hospital, Gail Carlyle at Glace Bay General Hospital, Peggy Bonnar at Glace Bay Community Hospital and Eileen Moore at New Waterford Consolidated Hospital.

The three-year diploma program was reduced to two years in 1969 with increased emphasis on theoretical preparation. Some schools closed, others amalgamated and the need for a nursing degree program was identified. Many graduates of nursing diploma programs became involved in distance education leading to nursing degrees. The local continuing education committee led a strong movement to develop a nursing degree program at Cape Breton University. Groundwork by Drs. Ora MacManus, Donald Dunbar, Bill Reid and Mr. Sheldon MacInnes, along with many others, eventually led to the joint Cape Breton University/St. FX Bachelor of Science in Nursing degree established in 1999.

For those entering the profession, the BSc degree became mandatory in 2000. For decades, there have been questions regarding the best balance of education and clinical experience. Nurses today are expected to coordinate plans of care, provide leadership in administrative roles, make critical client care decisions, provide education and do research.

## THE CAP AND UNIFORM

For at least 100 years, the nurse's white cap and uniform were the symbols of the nursing profession. Nurses wore them with pride and honour, because to them it represented not only the occupation, but the hospital, position and qualifications of the person who wore it. During the last 40 years or so, the uniform—or lack thereof—has sparked a minor controversy in the profession.

In their discussion on the nurse's cap, the Canadian Museum of Civilization cited many reasons that caps, along with the rest of uniforms, began to disappear in the 1970s. One of the main reasons was that nursing was becoming more professionalized and nurses wanted to identify with other professionals who wore no uniform. When hospitals employed nursing assistants, technicians and other groups, the authority of the nurse's cap began to erode.

In her article, "Nurses' Cap and Uniform: In Vogue or Obsolete," Associate Professor E. MacFarlane of the Department of Nursing at St. Francis Xavier University asks: "What other professional person has to be instructed about what to wear to work?"

She went on to say there are those who argue that the white uniform was very helpful to identify staff to patients, visitors and other health professionals. As will be seen from the variety of opinions expressed in this book, some people still argue the pros and cons about the uniform and caps today.

In the 1980s, nurses who worked in specialized units, such as psychiatry, no longer wore white uniforms, because research studies indicated they interfered with positive interpersonal relationships with clients/patients.

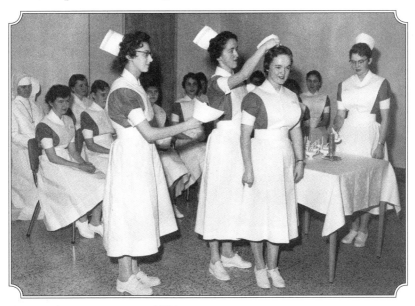

A capping ceremony, 1959.

Between 1960 and 1980, the cap began to lose its symbolic meaning of achievement. The apprentice system of hospital education, with progress through the ranks, no longer dominated nursing education. Universities and community colleges eventually replaced hospital-based schools of nursing.

In addition, although male nurses have always worn uniforms like other nurses, they have never worn caps.

## MODERN NURSING ISSUES

There has been a marked increase in the number of married nurses, males and representatives of ethnic minorities entering the profession. Nursing practitioners are now working in Cape Breton and their numbers are increasing. They are accepted, appreciated and fully utilized.

The role of the registered nurse is constantly expanding. Key issues such as workloads, absenteeism, educational opportunities and scope of practice have existed for decades. With all the advancements in technology and consequent changes in health care services, a fundamental question remains to be answered by the various stakeholders who have an interest in the direction of nursing as a profession. That question is: Are we providing the range and depth of preparation required by professional nurses to fulfill changing roles?

# FEATURED GRADUATES

## ST. JOSEPH'S HOSPITAL SCHOOL OF NURSING, GLACE BAY

Christina (MacDonald) MacIntyre, 1931                26
Margaret (Marchand) Cusack, 1944                    177
Dr. Simone Roach, 1947                               32
Jock Crosby, 1950                                    40
Caroline (Gromick) Paruch, 1956                      93
Betty (MacLellan) Dowe, 1957                         51
Janice Ferguson, 1964                               165
Judith (Ferguson) Gillis, 1965                      167
Gloria (Matheson) LeBlanc, 1970                     170

## GLACE BAY GENERAL HOSPITAL SCHOOL OF NURSING, GLACE BAY

Norma (MacKinnon) MacDonald, 1932                   28
Effie (MacDougall) Ormiston, 1934                   30
Jean (MacInnis) Hemsworth, 1945                     35
Gladys (Philips) Smith, 1946                        37
Geraldeen (Butler) Collins, 1951                    41
Anita (Skinner) Cousins, 1951                       44
Marion (MacLean) Hopkins, 1951                      46
Lenora Brewster, 1956                               48
Dr. Marion (Atkinson) MacIntosh, 1957               95
Jim Struthers, 1957                                 98
Alice (MacLean) Freeman, 1958                      159
Judy (Burden) Price, 1967                           53

## NEW WATERFORD GENERAL HOSPITAL SCHOOL OF NURSING, NEW WATERFORD

Emma (MacLean) MacDonald, 1940   58
Sister Barbara Muldoon, 1941   60
Irene (Herve) MacMillan, 1946   62
Eleanor (Morrison) Burke, 1946   64

## SYDNEY CITY HOSPITAL SCHOOL OF NURSING, SYDNEY

Rita (Jones) Smith, 1930   155
Grace (Whalen) Bonnar, 1934   74
Marion (Mitchell) MacDonald, 1937   77
Elsie (Dakai) Percy, 1941   79
Laura (Watts) MacKinnon, 1952   67
Lynne (Walker) Clarke, 1954   88
Shirley MacDonald, 1957   100
Tina (Matthews) Waters, 1960   160
Phyllis Ball, 1965   110
Thelma (Timmons) Grant, 1972   139

## ST. RITA HOSPITAL SCHOOL OF NURSING, SYDNEY

Carole Ravanello, 1962   108
Heather LeBlanc, 1970   172
Regina (Donovan) Williams, 1980   152

## HAMILTON SCHOOL OF NURSING AND ST. ELIZABETH'S HOSPITAL SCHOOL OF NURSING, NORTH SYDNEY

Betty Cordeau (Elizabeth), 1949   85
Natalie Wilkie, 1952   113
Irene (Stephenson) Funge, 1955   116
Kathleen Stephenson, 1955   118
Marilyn Morrison-Foley, 1956   120
Mary (Cleary) MacIssac, 1956   122
Tula (Mancini) Gouthro, 1956   123
Ann (Goss) Robinson, 1957   125
Amelia (Sylliboy) Jesty, 1958   127

Ann Marie (Day) (Grandy) Steele, 1958 130
Ann (Campbell) D'Andrea, 1960 101
Francis (Doucette) McIntyre, 1960 104
Jane (DeLeskie) Jessome, 1961 132
Vi (Mancini) Sampson, 1962 179
Ethel (Squarey) Cluett, 1963 135
Alfreda Douglas, 1965 137
Sharon (Donovan) Williams, 1966 150

## OFF-ISLAND NURSING SCHOOLS

Jessie (Kavanaugh) Curtis, Boston City Hospital, 1916 143
Hannah (MacDonald) Matheson,
 Massachusetts State Infirmary, 1931 145
Emily (MacLean) MacLeod, Salvation Army Grace Maternity,
 Halifax, 1935 147
Roberta (MacMillan) Cameron, Halifax Infirmary, 1945 157
Albert Orrell, Nova Scotia Hospital, Dartmouth, 1945 80
Edna (Farquhar) MacDougall, Jeffrey Hale Hospital,
 Quebec City, 1949 82
Clotilda (Coward) (Douglas) Yakimchuk, Nova Scotia Hospital,
 Dartmouth, 1954 90
Sister Veronica Matthews, St. Martha's
 Hospital, Antigonish, 1961 106
Betty Jane Cameron, McGill University, Montreal, 1961 162
Mary Lee (Waters) Morrison, Victoria General Hospital,
 Halifax, 1962 160
Claire (Roach) Timmons, St. Francis Xavier University,
 Antigonish, 1970 69
Mary (Chisholm) Fleck, Mount Wachusett College,
 Gardner, Massachusetts, 1976 174

# GRADUATE REFLECTIONS
# AND LOCAL HIGHLIGHTS

# GLACE BAY

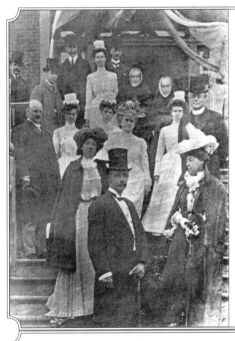

First graduating class from St. Joseph's Hospital School of Nursing, Glace Bay. Earl and Countess Gray in the foreground; Annie (MacAskill) MacAulay at top centre. Courtesy Donna Young.

1902: The first nursing school in Cape Breton opened at St. Joseph's Hospital in Glace Bay. The first class of nurses graduated in 1905. In 1915, the Sisters of St. Martha took over the hospital.

1920: The Department of Health hired nurses to work in town schools.

1927: St. Joseph's celebrated its Silver Jubilee. A staff residence was built in 1932. In 1939 a new wing and a TB unit opened.

# CHRISTINA (MACDONALD) MACINTYRE

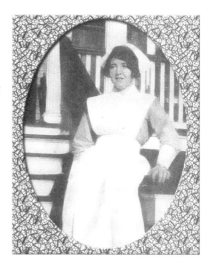

*Christina graduated from St. Joseph's School of Nursing in Glace Bay in 1931. She began her career as a general duty nurse at St. Joseph's Hospital but, like all nurses of her era, had to leave the hospital after marriage. Christina went on to nurse for various local agencies and ended her career as a night supervisor in a nursing school residence. She shares joyful and vivid memories of a full career.*

I became a nurse because I care so much for people. I had a large family and, being the oldest girl, I helped look after the siblings. Classmates were like family as we lived together and trained together for three years. There were nine in my class and I am the only one remaining alive.

When we were in our first year, we wore a long starched blue dress with white apron, shoes and hat. They had to be spotless. Each shift we had to line up in front of the supervisor and be inspected. Upon graduation we received a white dress uniform and a black band for our nursing cap. Today I find you cannot tell the difference between the nurses, cleaners and Licenced Practical Nurses. Very rarely do you see someone with their cap and white uniform.

I worked general duty on the main floor after graduation. I also worked in the accident ward, medical ward and obstetrics. The hospital always had everything we needed for the care of the miners after the many accidents. You were paid $4 for a 12-hour shift. There was a detox unit in the basement. Many times, community notables would be sneaked down and their identity kept secret. Sometimes the detox patients would sneak out and we would have to go find them, especially the notables. It was done very quickly. Most times, the patients were only wearing a hospital gown.

Once, I was cleaning up a man's clothes off the floor and here was his artificial leg. It made me so nervous I had to go and have someone come in with me. There were also the times when you had to take a patient to the morgue. The elevator was very shaky when it first started … one time a man's arm fell out of bed and hit my side.

I left nursing at the hospital when I was married as you were not given work in the hospital if you were married. I went on to work for the Victorian Order of Nurses, Social Services, Metropolitan Life, Public Health. You were paid $5 a shift for private duty. I worked a 24-hour shift and was provided a cot to sleep on, but you would never be able to sleep because the patients would keep you awake talking. I was paid $10 a month at Social Services and driven around by chauffeur to homes for prenatal and postnatal visits. I also did postnatal visits for Metropolitan Life and sometimes looked after seniors or elderly. As a public health nurse, you were always working, even though you were off, as the community relied heavily on you and often people were sent to your house. If their condition was serious, I took them to the hospital.

As a nurses' residence night supervisor I worked 4-to-12. I was responsible for ensuring the nurses came back by 10 p.m. curfew. If they came in late, I would talk to them rather than discipline them. If it was a serious incident, I would report it to my supervisor. If the nurses did not return before the end of my shift, I would write down their names for my relief. The girls used to sneak out the windows after the lights

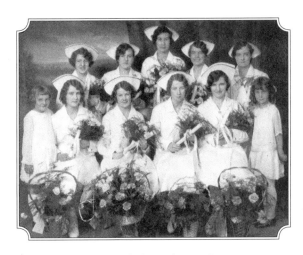

St. Joseph's Hospital class of 1931. Front row: Monica Morley (flower girl), Jessie MacIntosh, Helen Murphy, Sadie V. MacKinnon, Margaret MacMahon, Madeline MacDonald Hines (flower girl). Second row: Christina (MacDonald) MacIntyre, Ellen O'Connor, Margaret Ann Gillis, Florence Bosh, Margaret Cameron.

were out or have other girls distract me after I made my rounds so the others could sneak out. I laughed at their tricks; it was as fun and enjoyable as the rest of my career. This was my most relaxing position, from 1959 to 1969.

Over time, I saw nursing classes getting larger and larger and, with constant advances in medicine, the nurses were becoming much more knowledgeable, but with classes so large, I wonder if they have as many close personal relationships as we had. Nurses today have better relationships with the doctors.

## NORMA (MACKINNON) MACDONALD

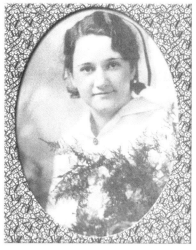

*Norma graduated from Glace Bay General Hospital School of Nursing in 1932 and completed postgraduate training in Montreal. She worked in administration in Glace Bay until her marriage in 1944. Norma was away from nursing for twenty-seven years while she raised her family. She resumed her nursing career at age fifty-two and worked another twenty years as an obstetrical nurse. Norma retired in 1972 with fond memories of patient care.*

Growing up I always solved a lot of problems for everybody, so my mother and father had decided that they were going to make a lawyer out of me because I was good at solving problems (we had five girls and one boy and they were all professionals and all did what they wanted to do). Anyway, when my father got sick my older sister was a nurse. She came back home to look after him. I don't know what he had. I remember he was unconscious; he had not spoken for days. I washed his face and cleaned out his eyes. I was fourteen. He opened his eyes and said: "Oh Norma." He recovered from that and after he got better, he said to my mother: "You know, we always said we would make a lawyer out of Norma, but it would be a shame because she is a born nurse." So they suggested I go in and be a nurse, and I loved it.

I went into training in 1928 and I was out a year, I had pleurisy. When I went back, I went into the next class so I graduated in 1932.

I always enjoyed training, it was a really nice experience because I was fond of people and all seemed to like me for some reason or another. I went from one department to another. I lived in the old residence. The housemother had a big dog. A lot of them did not like her but I did. When I would come home with a box of chocolates from a date, I would always treat her. I would go in and she would keep me to find out all of the news. I was a little bit late (you had to be on time), but she would never say anything to me because I would treat her with chocolates.

I worked at the old Glace Bay General for about six months or so after I graduated, but then I went to Montreal to the Children's Hospital and took postgraduate work. When I finished the course in Montreal they invited me to stay on staff, but I couldn't do that because my mother was ill and I wanted to come home and look after her and I did. After she died, I went over to the General and was supervisor on second floor. That was in 1933 and I worked there until the later part of 1944 and got married. When you got married, you went home.

So I was home for twenty-seven years and in all that time I was a second mother for everybody in the community. I had a daughter that trained at the General, she graduated in 1952. One day the Director of Nursing said: "We have a refresher course for all of the old nurses, I wonder about your mother." I thought it would be very nice to get back into the heart of it so I did. I got hired and was on first floor working on the charts and the time sheets. Shortly after that they were looking for an obstetrical nurse. I said: "I guess babies come the same way as they did twenty-seven years ago," and that I would go. I stayed there for twenty years. It was fun.

When I had to do the recording of the charts, the greatest difference I saw after twenty-seven years was the chart. As far as nursing care, it was the same nursing care I was giving when I was twenty-five as I was doing when I was fifty, but the charts were a little different. I was never in a hurry, if three o'clock came and there were things to be done, I would stay and do it.

The bedside nursing seems to be left to the practical nurses and I don't think the regular nurses fuss over the patients anymore. Maybe they would like to but the paperwork seems to be more important. I would like for the nurses to look after the patients and sit down and be able to talk to them. I did that for a lady and she was my friend afterward. She had a Down Syndrome baby and nobody wanted to tell her, they waited until I came on duty to tell her. I went down into the room and sat down to talk to her and I told her and compared her baby to others with the same situation, how they got along and enjoyed life and whatnot. We became great friends and to this day she said how thankful she was that I had talked to her when other people turned their heads in the other direction and did not tell her anything.

I think it is disgraceful the way nurses look today because when you got your cap, you were so proud to wear it and now they don't wear them anymore. There is one nurse at the Regional Hospital that still wears her cap and every time I see her I tell her she looks nice. Now, with the flowery tops you don't know if it is the one scrubbing the floor or the one that is bringing the food, or the one that is looking after the sick.

## EFFIE (MacDOUGALL) ORMISTON

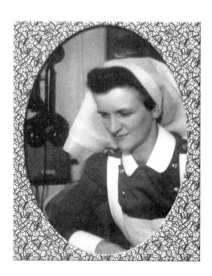

*Effie graduated from Glace Bay General in 1934 in the midst of the Great Depression. She worked in Montreal for a year and returned to Glace Bay General where she worked until she joined the war effort in 1942. Effie retired in 1950 to marry and raise a family but has strong memories of her training, nursing in a mining community and her experiences during the Depression and World War II.*

When I was about fourteen, I belonged to a group who were taken to the hospital just to show us how things were. I thought this was just marvelous and wanted to be a nurse from then on. I had to wait a year after high school to be old enough to enter. I found it hard work but really enjoyed the challenge. I was very lucky, as I didn't miss a day during the three years. Influenza and smallpox was going around at the time. When a patient left, you cleaned and disinfected the entire room, changed the drapes and cleaned the windows.

I remember we wore a blue dress with short sleeves that had a bib and apron. It was a great pride that in six months you could receive a cap and if you didn't receive your cap it was considered a setback. And then, when you were in the beginning of your third year, they gave you black velvet to put on your cap and show that you were a senior nurse, almost finished. And it was an honour to receive it. When I went to Montreal, I wore my Glace Bay General cap.

When I wrote the provincial exam, I was informed that I led the province and to me that was a great accomplishment in itself. It was a small training school and a 100-bed hospital, but we received very good training. They had so many mine accidents and so many cases that other hospitals might not have looked after. Unfortunately, when you finished the nursing program, it was the Great Depression and there was a lot of nurses, very few had jobs, especially in the hospitals.

So, I went to Montreal and worked at the Royal Victoria in gynecology and obstetrics. I went on to the Alexandra Hospital which looked after communicable diseases. Then I got a job looking after TB patients and I think it was $60 a month they paid. That was in 1936. I heard there was a position in the Glace Bay General as assistant night supervisor so I applied and was approved. I was also interested in blood counts and cross matching of blood. I went to the Saint John General Hospital to take blood chemistry. I was interested in the patient as a whole.

During the Great Depression, of course, there was a lot of illness and when you are a nurse in the neighbourhood you go ahead and help but you would never think of charging as the family could not afford it.

I stayed at the Glace Bay General for the rest of my career until the war came along. I joined in January of 1942 and served in England and Italy, then back to England and home. I looked after people with diphtheria, malaria, dysentery, TB, hepatitis and everything else. During the war, certain nurses were not allowed to enlist because it was felt they were so needed at home. The staff at Camp Hill remained there as they were really needed.

I felt I did a good job looking after sick people. I was very proud of my work. Relationships with patients, especially mine accidents, were heartbreaking and joyful. I wish I could only start all over again. I retired in 1950 because I decided to get married. It was important to stay with children, especially when they were small.

---

1938: The Glace Bay branch of the Victorian Order of Nurses was abandoned.

1941: Glace Bay General Hospital opened a new wing. A children's unit followed in 1943.

---

## DR. SIMONE ROACH

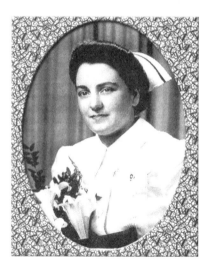

*D*r. Simone Roach graduated from St. Joseph's School of Nursing in 1944. In 1945, she entered the Sisters of St. Martha and was assigned to St. Martha's Hospital in Antigonish. She completed a Bachelor of Science at St. Francis Xavier University. Simone also completed a program in hospital administration in Toronto and then moved to Massachusetts to work in administration in an American nursing school. She completed her doctorate in the United States in 1970 and returned to St. FX to chair the Nursing Department. She later spent several years at Harvard, at St. Boniface Hospital, Winnipeg, and at St. Regis College, Toronto. Her writing and research on the philosophical foundations of human caring and spirituality have been presented internationally. Her passion for nursing, teaching and the future of her profession remains strong.

I worked for one year, believe it or not, as a school nurse at St. Agnes School in New Waterford. It was the whole school,

grades primary and up, in 1944-45 and I will never forget the
graciousness and the help I received from the public health nurse
from the region. Being a nurse was a way of caring for others.

After that year I entered the Sisters of St. Martha in Antigonish
and after two years, in 1947, I took first vows and was assigned
to St. Martha's Hospital as Supervisor of Obstetrics. In five or six
months, I was an expert! In those days it was not only Sisters, it
was typical of graduates to get such responsibility. I enjoyed it
very much. I became quite skilled and competent because I was
teaching as well as supervising. I did a diploma program at the
University of Toronto in clinical teaching and supervision in 1951.
I came back and taught at St. Martha's in the school and
eventually became director of the school. At the same time, I was
finishing my Bachelor of Science degree in nursing at St. FX.

In 1959, I returned to St. Joseph's Hospital in Glace Bay and taught
in the school of nursing for a year. Then I completed a year in
hospital administration at the University of Toronto, in 1960, and
worked in the school of nursing there. In 1961, we took over the
administration of a hospital in Lowell, Massachusetts, and I was
appointed coordinator for the school of nursing. During this time
I completed a master's degree in nursing at Boston University.
In 1967, I went to Washington, DC, to pursue a doctorate, which I
received in 1970 and at that time came to St. FX and took over as
chair of the Department of Nursing.

My philosophy of nursing was embedded and integrated into
everything I taught. My preference for teaching when I went to
St. FX was the first-year course. I wanted to teach the students
when they come into nursing before they are spoiled by any of
us, to reinforce what I believed to be the motivation of students
entering nursing: enthusiasm and the desire to care for people.
One of the first points that I would make with the first-year
university student would be when we speak about the diploma
graduates or the degree graduates or nursing assistant graduates,
we are not talking good, better, best but rather about the need to
design programs that prepared nurses for specific roles. I make
no apologies whatsoever for the quality of nursing education I
received from the diploma schools; most graduates, I'm sure,
would say the same thing.

Today, however, with the changes in health care in hospitals and in the community, it is not possible for a hospital diploma program to prepare a professional nurse for the required knowledge and skills. Nursing is more than the acquisition of basic skills—as extremely important as these are—to be professionally prepared, to develop an expanded critical thinking capacity, the nurse needs a foundation in the sciences and humanities. This is a foundation a hospital diploma program cannot give. That is not to say the diploma program has not made a great contribution to nursing over the years … the whole climate, culture, everything was so different to what it is now, it is difficult to make comparisons. It is only the people who were in nursing schools of that time who would understand that these schools provided most of the services in the hospitals.

Now you will sometimes hear persons, in all good faith and in concern for the status of the health system with respect to staffing, saying we should go back to hospital diploma programs. I think that would be most unfortunate, not because we weren't well prepared in the past, but because a diploma program cannot prepare a nurse for required roles today and for the future. That is a comment I feel strongly about. To me the purpose of the degree program in nursing is to prepare practitioners—not administrators, not supervisors but good clinical practitioners—in nursing at the first level.

I left St. FX in 1979 to do work on a Canadian Nurses Association project, the development of a code of ethics. I studied ethics in 1980-81 at Harvard Divinity School. Then I came back to St. FX and was there until 1986 at which time I facilitated two senior seminars. One was on trends in health care, the other was on research applied to nursing.

My definition, my concept, I should say, of health is grounded in philosophical language but out of that came the concept of health as peace, harmony and integration within the person, within the family and within the community. For me, nursing has always been a call of service to others, the professionalization of the human capacity to care.

# Jean (MacInnis) Hemsworth

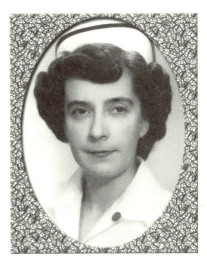

*Jean graduated from Glace Bay General in 1945. She continued her studies in nursing education at the University of Toronto. Jean provided bedside care for a few years in Toronto, but returned to Cape Breton to teach nursing. In 1963, after more study, Jean moved into hospital administration, a career she enjoyed until her retirement in 1992. Her memories span almost fifty years of health care in Cape Breton.*

Teaching or nursing: I had a bit of a problem deciding which. My mother encouraged me to go into teaching, but I decided that I wanted to be a nurse. It always appealed to me. I always liked working with people.

I was an only girl in the family and between living in residence and all the girls, it was certainly a real experience, and it was all kinds of fun. My brother was a male nurse. We graduated in the same class but there was no future in it so he went back to university and got his chartered accounting degree. He loved nursing. He used to say even though he had a good job, the job he loved most was when he studied nursing.

I took my three-year general duty at the Glace Bay General and then I became an RN and went to the University of Toronto and took my nursing education. I went to Toronto in 1946. My bedside nursing experience was there. I remember one teenager that I had as a patient and he had cancer in the leg and I can remember how terrible that was and the amount of care he required. He was only seventeen. I remember another woman who was twenty-eight; she had cancer and she was so irritable. We were young and we did not understand. You know when you are eighteen and someone is twenty-eight, they are quite old.

When I came home, I started to teach until 1963. As a nurse, I think preparing the students for nursing and seeing them gloating and doing well, that I think was satisfying. Then I became the director of the School of Nursing and continued in that for eight years and left and went to the Point Edward Hospital as Assistant Superintendent of Nursing. In that time, they established the affiliated program in TB nursing for student nurses. I combined both the instructor job and assistant superintendent job. Then I decided there was greater challenge in the acute care hospital so I was asked to come back to teaching.

I decided to go for something else so I went for the two-year HOM course in the Hospital of Administration. In 1963, the job came up as administrator. I was not terribly interested in it because of the responsibilities, but I was approached to consider it so I did, and did it for twenty-nine years.

Until 1959, the hospital was supported exclusively by the miners through a check-off system and you had to operate off that. My budget at that time was about $300,000 and when I left it was $11 million.

I took part, of course, in the organizations that were associated while I was in nursing. I belonged to the Registered Nurses Association, I was president in the area for awhile and I was on the board of examiners for the registration of nursing in Nova Scotia for ten years. In administration, I achieved fellowship status, that was a seven-year thing. I served as a regional representative for the Atlantic provinces for health care administrators and I was on the board of the Nova Scotia Association of Health Organizations for three years. I was president of the association in Cape Breton for a total of three years.

You were responsible for all the departments of the hospital and each one has a head so you go through the head. In a hospital of our size, we had 231 employees roughly; if you took the part-timers you would have more than that. I liked personal contact with the employees. I found it hard with nursing because there were so many of them and there were so many part-time. You are responsible for the public relations of the hospital and you have to sell yourself to the community.

I would do it over again even though you don't have time for yourself. I always had a live-in housekeeper. My husband was great at that too but it is very time consuming. I would do it over again, it is extremely interesting.

I retired in 1992. I was sixty-five. I had grown tired of it and they were talking about merging hospitals and it became a hot issue. I had been involved in it and it just reached the point that I had enough.

## GLADYS (PHILIPS) SMITH

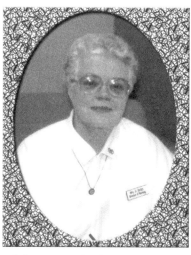

*Gladys graduated from Glace Bay General in 1946 and began a long career in that community. She also enjoyed an active role in her professional association locally and provincially, serving as Chair of the Cape Breton Branch of the Registered Nurses Association of Nova Scotia from 1967 to 1969, provincial president from 1976 to 1978 and on the board of both the RNANS and the Canadian Nurses Association. She retired in 1992. Gladys was on the front lines, witnessing decades of change in the health care system and shares her memories and insight.*

I was a product of the three-year nursing diploma program offered by the Glace Bay General Hospital School of Nursing, a public hospital-based apprenticeship program where the students provided the nursing care for the hospital patients in exchange for board and an education in nursing. My nursing education took place during the immediate postwar period. The atmosphere was somewhat militaristic in its discipline; students rising to stand at attention at the nursing stations, on stairways until their superiors passed. The nurses residence was a modern and attractive facility. Three classes of nursing students were living in residence at one time. The school used a proctor system for monitoring student behaviour, a senior student appointed to monitor the orderliness, noise level, to see that all students were accounted for and that lights were out at 11 p.m.

I enjoyed my nursing experience from day one. I appreciated the advantages of living in residence and of working closely with a group preparing to enter the same field. Probationary students attended classes in basic nursing care and procedures before being assigned to provide patient care as junior student nurses. All students were identified by a name bar fastened to the bib, but levels of achievement were identified by the colour of the band worn on the cap. Student nurses were rotated through each of the nursing units. The obstetrics and pediatric units were very busy services. Ten to twenty babies in the nursery were not unusual. A polio epidemic in 1947 turned the medical wards on floor one into an isolation unit.

This was before prepaid government hospital and medical insurance programs were in place. Despite a modest weekly payroll check-off system in the mines and steel plant, hospitals in the area were hard pressed to meet their commitments. There were periods when boards had to turn to banks for loans to meet expenses. The nursing program was an inexpensive, cost effective method of meeting the nursing care needs of patients from 1946 to the 1970s. Area doctors held regular afternoon and evening clinics and made house calls, so there was little demand for out-patient services. In 1959 and 1964, with the introduction of the Hospital Insurance and Medical Care Act, the focus shifted to the organization of health care. Issues centered on availability of services, replacement of outdated hospitals, preparation and increase in numbers of doctors, nurses and a variety of professionals. With the prepaid government health service, registered nursing staff were hired on the hospital units to replace the service component in the nursing education program. The focus shifted to an emphasis on the theory of nursing with a supporting nursing practice/experience component. Lengths of stay in hospitals were examined and gradually reduced for specific populations. Student nurses were unable to get the required experience in the home-based hospital and affiliate programs were arranged at the Grace Maternity Hospital, Point Edward Hospital and the Kentville Sanatorium. After review in the late 1960s, the diploma schools moved into the two-year nursing program. In Cape Breton, the three-year schools closed in swift succession; New Waterford and Glace Bay in 1970 and then St. Elizabeth's on the Northside. The two schools in Sydney, St. Rita's and Sydney City, continued to provide nursing practitioners, graduates of the two-year diploma program for the Cape Breton area for the next fifteen years.

The 1970s and 1980s were the years of plenty in Canada's health system, a system increasing in complexity and cost. Under the guidance of the RNANS, in the early 1970s, collective bargaining for nursing was promoted to improve the benefits offered to the membership. The first provincial strike began in June of 1975.

Nursing diploma programs began to be phased out in favour of preparation of nurses at the degree level. By 1996, the two schools in Sydney closed, prior to the opening of the new Regional Hospital. Cape Breton now had no ready supply of Island nurses to provide relief or replace normal staff attrition.

It's been more than twelve years since I retired. For months afterward, I experienced feelings of separation anxiety and sadness. I missed the associations with "my team," the people I worked alongside for so many years, the variety of experiences that a changing health care service provides and the sense of satisfaction that comes when the organization you serve functions smoothly. There was always the problem-solving role to challenge and stimulate interest. The nursing I was familiar with in the '60s, '70s and '80s was a soul-satisfying field.

The wise and experienced nurse knows well that she is always responsible for her actions, regardless of the written order. The nurse is the caregiver, the observer, the listener and advocate for the patient, speaking out in the interests of her client. She is also responsible for ensuring that her nursing unit is patient friendly. Nursing is the glue that holds the health system together.

Nursing and health care continue to be in a state of flux. I worry that a shortage of nurses to meet the changing needs of today's health care system may have a lasting effect, where disillusioned nurses may impart such a negative view of the frustrations of their situations that prospective students may turn away from nursing. As for me, I am grateful that I was blessed to have experienced the best years Canada's health care system had to offer. The people I grew to know, the experiences that crossed my path, have given my life a richness I could never have otherwise known.

## JOCK CROSBY

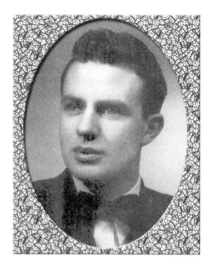

*Jock graduated from St. Joseph's Hospital School of Nursing, Glace Bay, in 1950. He worked in a large Toronto Hospital for five years before making a career change. Jock recalls the differences between male and female nursing roles in the 1950s and the changes in hospital care over the decades.*

I have no idea why I became a nurse. I was planning on medicine and it just didn't work out. There were two of us males graduating. I have all good training memories. I did not stay in the nurses' residence. I stayed in what they called the interning room. That was on the second floor of the old wing of the hospital, a very big room. They didn't have interns anymore. We were in all departments but obstetrics, or anything looking after women. What I mostly did instead of obstetrics was prostate and urinary problems. Now, I think they do all of it. In 1947, that was a no-no.

We had a ward with about sixteen patients in it. All male, we were assigned certain patients. Plus, when I was in training, we had to do the cleaning of the wards and the floors. Mop the floors and do the lockers. When someone left or died, we had to carbolize the beds.

They treated me a little differently. You were kind of special, I guess, kind of separate from the rest. We didn't have to keep hours or anything like that. We didn't have to be in at ten o'clock. We could come in whenever and the other nurses had to be in at ten. We would come back after ten and I would go in the front door. One of the sisters would be at the front desk watching for people, for nurses sneaking in. I would go in and keep her very busy with all the chatting we did while they snuck through the window downstairs. Sometimes they were caught, but I was there to distract her. We had a very good relationship. She liked the news so I would make up some news.

There were a lot of nice people in our class. I kept friendly with them all and I still attend the anniversaries that they have. The hospital in Toronto was large. I was supervisor of a ward where they only did back surgery. They were all workers' compensation cases, mostly foreign people. They had the surgery done and they were kept in bed for so long, not up the next day and walking. And we'd have them for perhaps two months. Then they would recuperate and get physiotherapy and things like that. It was just a daily routine of washing, bathing and giving them medication, making up the beds. We were never allowed to start an IV like they can now. We were allowed to give out meds. Otherwise it was just bedside manner, seeing that they were comfortable.

Our uniforms were just white pants and a top. It came over and buttoned down the side. There were no caps or anything. I think the current changes in uniforms is unprofessional. I'd be over there at the [Glace Bay] General and I wouldn't know who was who. One day I was asking somebody where to get something and she said: "I'm sorry but I'm the cleaning lady." It is definitely a problem now—you don't know who you are talking to, who's looking after you or who's in the room.

I retired from nursing in 1955. I just thought I needed another field to work in and it came up. When I was in Toronto, I was making $75 a month. I was paying $5 a week for room and board. After I came back from Toronto I did some private duty. I worked over in the General. I worked at St. Rita's in Sydney until I got this other job for $240 a month. So I went and worked for the provincial government until 1963, then I was hired by the federal government. I retired in 1992. It was a money thing. It wasn't that I didn't like nursing.

## GERALDEEN (BUTLER) COLLINS

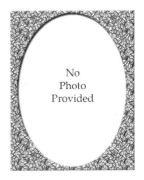

No
Photo
Provided

*Geraldeen graduated from Glace Bay General in 1951 and worked in maternity, private duty, clinics and industrial nursing before beginning a career as an Enterstomal Therapist (medical care to patients with colostomies, ileostomies and urostomies). She especially enjoyed the opportunities specialized nursing gave her to develop relationships with her patients. Geraldeen's commitment to patient care and her love of her profession made her reluctant to retire and happy to return when needed.*

When I was very young, I had my tonsils out and I was very impressed with the nurse. I always remembered that. It was close to home and you never had to go away anywhere. When you are in the middle of six children, finances were tight because Dad worked at the steel plant and Mom didn't work. It was free. I don't remember paying anything or did we pay for one year? If so, it was very little. My aunt was one of the ones who made the uniforms.

We lived in residence. When we first started, we were in the basement and it was a big room. There were eight of us. We had bunk beds and we shared great memories, our sorrows, cried together, laughed together. One of the bad things might have been the ten o'clock curfew. If you did not make it back on time, you could be locked out and suffer the consequences, like lose some of your privileges. I trained in Glace Bay, but I lived on St. Peter's Road in Sydney. When we first began our program, we would have the weekends off. I would come home, but if it was stormy, I would not be able to get back.

After graduation, you went wherever you wanted and I applied to Royal Avenue Maternity because I wanted to work in the nursery more than maternity, but there you worked in both places because it was integrated. I enjoyed working maternity, but at this time young married nurses were not allowed to work in maternity. I did some private duty and relief nursing at Glace Bay General Hospital and from there I went to work in the Bay Medical Clinic. I was assigned mostly to an area where I did dressings. I gave injections whether it was allergy shots, penicillin injections or whatever.

From there I went into industrial nursing where I had my own little trailer. If someone were to get something in their eye, they would have to report to me, or if they had a sprain. It was a great experience. I got to climb the tower. A young guy froze when he got to the top and no amount of convincing by the guys that he could come down so I had to go up there and come down with him. The worst thing that happened was when a man fell and died, now that was a bad experience.

Coming out of church one day, someone mentioned that the
hospital was looking for an Enterstomal Therapist. So I thought
about it and applied. Because the job was sponsored by the
Canadian Cancer Society out of Halifax, I had to go there for the
interview. When I got there, there was a young girl who was also
waiting to be interviewed for a job in Cape Breton. As an older
nurse, I thought, "Yew, I might as well go home now," but I got it.
I went off to the clinic so it was difficult coming back and saying
okay, this is my specialty. Some of the doctors would look at you
and say: "Well what do you think you could tell us that we haven't
done?" I was just able to bring them up to date on the newer
procedures.

To be able to help someone adjust to the fact that there was a big
change in their body, I mean a lot of people figure they should
go home and die. Today the ostomy pouches are sophisticated
as opposed to years ago when they had rubber ones that would
remind you of bicycle tires, rubbery and thick. Actually they
weren't using those when I was in Cleveland receiving my
training, but they had them in the archives so we could see them
and know how they started and what they have progressed to.

I would feel badly because I would go in and see the patient and
tell them what kind of surgery they were going to have, if they
have stoma, and explain all this to them and you would hope
that everything goes well. I would have different sizes and types
of stomas so they would know. There was this one gentleman
that was totally upset, he was going to be done as an emergency.
Luckily I had been at the hospital when he was admitted and he
was very concerned about how big the stoma was going to be.
I said no, it wouldn't be and he went off to the OR and I went
back to one of the hospitals. The next time I was in, I went to
see him and there was the stoma and it was large. I nearly cried
and you can't let on that you are shocked, you have to keep your
expressions to yourself. The patients appreciated the fact that I
could spend more time with them, not like the regular nurses,
because this was my specialty. I had a better relationship with my
patients, being able to see them after they went home and you got
to know them as they would come in and see me for their follow-
up visits. If they brought their son or daughter, you got to know
them, too. That made for a good relationship.

There were not many male nurses early in my career, but later on there were. They were always very professional, very considerate of the female patient and you never felt embarrassed with them around. They looked after more of the male patients than they do today. I mean, today they are more equal in the eyes of the people.

I retired when I turned 65 and had to, there was no ifs, maybes or buts. Previous to that you were allowed if the hospital wanted you and you were healthy, but a few months before I turned 65, the law was passed and it was "Out!" Luckily, they had not replaced me right away and the doctors kicked up a fuss so I was called back. You don't miss the work, you miss the people. Before you retire, they talk to you about finances and stuff, but they never talked to you about your emotion.

## ANITA (SKINNER) COUSINS

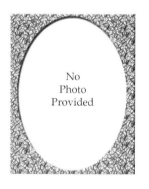

No Photo Provided

*A nita graduated from Glace Bay General in 1951 and began her career in her home town of Inverness. She traded small town life for the excitement of an emergency room in Toronto. She eventually moved to Halifax where she worked in the operating room in the specialized field of neurosurgery. Anita nursed part-time while raising her family and taught as a surgical nurse in a dental school for a year. She retired in 1970 to concentrate on raising her children, but has remained active and interested in health care.*

I never, ever thought of doing anything else. My mom said I used to bandage my dolls when I was a little girl. I knew from scratch. There was no doubt in my mind and I don't regret it one bit.

Our nursing training was very strict, everything we did was supervised. If we had to do a dressing, we'd be supervised three times and by this time, I guess they figured we would know how to do it properly. We had excellent instructors. We got along fine and I loved my classmates. We had a reunion a couple of years ago and we had a great time. I still keep in touch with about a half a dozen of them.

After graduation, I went to my hometown in Inverness, worked there for a year or so and decided maybe we should try the green fields far away in Toronto. I worked at the emergency department up there. We had to be in charge of the operating room while we were on duty. Then, when I came back to Nova Scotia, I decided I'd do OR. I worked with the only neurosurgeon in Nova Scotia, very specialized, the instruments, the whole procedure. Then I got married and had two sons and that was it for awhile.

I went back and did some general surgery. I stopped working again and went back and did a stint at the dental school as the surgery nurse, teaching these techniques to dental students. I taught at this particular time because they needed someone with OR experience. That only lasted about a year. I'd rather be right in the middle of it than teach, though. We worked hard. In extreme cases we would go down to the wards to see the patients post-op—especially in neurosurgery. I remember being in the OR all night. I did two patients and they both died. Now that was really hard, but then there is satisfaction in other things. In the operating room, it is a team. Everything relies on the other person, from day one.

I stopped working when my son was born and then I went back for a year and a half. I was sort of up and down and never stuck with my career for any length of time. I did some volunteering and things like that to help out in the neighbourhood.

People really, I think, respect nurses more than they ever did. I guess I could say I'm an advisor. I live in a condominium in Halifax. Three times I've been in an ambulance taking my neighbours. They would call me. One night, I thought this woman was having a stroke and I took her. People depend on me when they know I'm a nurse. But I haven't worked for years. I did some volunteer work at Victoria General Hospital and it was just nice to be back in that environment.

I wish it would go back to training schools. I think they would be much more at ease with patients instead of coming out of classes and all of a sudden you're there with a very sick person. It must be hard. Years ago you started from day one, just doing little things, tidying up the bedside table. You always had bedside contact. But I agree with patients going home sooner from the hospital. I think they feel much better at home rather than staying in hospital for a prolonged time. Home is where you are most relaxed.

## MARION (MacLean) HOPKINS

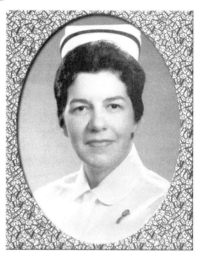

*Marion graduated from Glace Bay General in 1951 and worked in the operating room at the Victoria General Hospital in Halifax for seventeen years. She then moved back to Cape Breton to teach in the certified nursing assistant program. She officially retired in 1987, but returned to teach the final year in the New Waterford Hospital's training program and to work relief in Glace Bay. Marion's last nursing role was at the forefront of home care in eastern Nova Scotia. Her memories include the drama of a big city operating room, the rewards of teaching and the early days of community care.*

I wanted to be a nurse right from the start. My cousin, who graduated in 1945, was my role model. I used to love to see her in uniform. They were good times in the residence at night. We were still just kids and we shared things because we only got $7 a month. That's what we got for the first two years. And I think our senior year we got $12. And out of that money you had to buy your toothpaste and deodorant and your nylons. You cleaned the floors when you were a student nurse. You mopped the floors and cleaned the beds and did the housekeeping as well as the nursing.

You know in training days, we really respected the head nurse: I wouldn't say we were afraid, but I guess it was respect. It was cautious respect. I mean, you went out in the morning, or in the evening, depending on what shift you were on, and you stood at the desk with the other nursing staff to hear the report. You were inspected whether you wanted to be or not. Whether you knew it or not, the head nurse was sizing you up to see if your shoes were clean and if your uniform was intact, or whatever. They ran a tight shift. And that's why we got such good training.

I did work at the hospital for a few months as assistant to the night supervisor. And then I went to Halifax to take a postgraduate course in operating room at the Halifax Infirmary. When I finished my course, I went directly to the VG hospital and I was there a total of seventeen years. I started out in general surgery. At one point, I was assistant OR supervisor. In the later part of my time there I became supervisor of chest and cardiovascular surgery in orthopedics. I was privileged to have been part of the team of the very first open heart surgery that was done in Nova Scotia. I loved the OR, I loved it.

I can remember when I went to the VG first. And I was very intimidated by all these big surgeries they were doing and all these rooms and these surgeons. I can remember one evening being in a room with all these strangers, it was just before we went off duty, and we were discussing the surgery that was going to take place the next day. And one of the doctors said: "Oh, we won't have to worry because Ms. MacLean will be here."

In 1967, they built the new wing at the VG. Just before it was to be opened (it was in the summer and I was off duty), everybody was called back. A plane had crashed in Newfoundland, a Czechoslovakian plane. They brought a lot of these people who were badly burned to the VG. And the ambulances were coming one after another. Many of them didn't survive. But they had to open—they had to put them in the new wing. The plastic surgeon and staff worked for forty-eight hours nonstop.

When I left the VG to come back to Cape Breton, I went to what they call now the community college, it was the vocational school then. Doing their clinical training for the certified nursing assistants, or what they call now the LPNs. And I was there for about thirteen years and decided it was time to retire. In fact I did in 1987. And that summer I received a call from the New Waterford Hospital because it was the final year they were training students. So I went for that final year to New Waterford and it was like a step back in time because their students lived in residence. And they had rules. They had to be in at ten, like I did. And their rooms were inspected every week.

So, I finished that year and was sitting home enjoying myself and they were setting up Nova Scotia home care in this area. I went to do that. It ended up being over a period of seven or eight years because it went from this area to include the whole of Cape Breton Island, Guysborough, Antigonish and Pictou counties. That was the last thing I did as a nurse and I enjoyed it so much because it was basic nursing.

We're always going to need nurses. I hope we can encourage more young people to go into nursing and to make it easier to get in. There are so many caring young people out there that want to be nurses. But it's so difficult for them now, it costs so much. When I trained it didn't cost us. We had to pay for our uniforms and pay for our books. But it was a different era. We were the staff of the hospital. Now it's a university degree and the cost is there. In one sense we've lost a lot by not having training schools. Lost a great deal. Is there an answer? If there is, I don't have it. I'm just hopeful. The nurses are the backbone of the hospital and that's fact.

1902-1952 St. Joseph's Hospital
Admissions – 121,796
Births – 14,296
Operations – 33,563
Hospital Days – 1,657,315

## LENORA BREWSTER

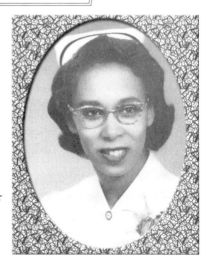

*Lenora graduated from Glace Bay General in 1956 and nursed in the area briefly before moving to the Nova Scotia Hospital. She studied psychiatric nursing in Massachusetts and worked in Montreal and later in corrections. Lenora remembers the prejudice she faced as a Black working woman in the 1950s and the challenges and rewards of specialized nursing.*

I finished high school and I had no idea what I wanted to do. My high school buddy was going into training. There were two or three more girls with us that decided we were all going in training. There was some difficulty getting into training in Cape

Breton, there was a lot of prejudice here. You could not get into the City Hospital or St. Rita's, none of the hospitals except New Waterford took Blacks in training. My father knew the brother of the superintendent of the Glace Bay General. I spoke to him and he said he will consider my application so I got into training there. On graduation, I was kind of fearful: "Now where am I going to work because if they don't want me training in their hospital, maybe they would not want me working there."

I started private duty at the Glace Bay General. From there I went to New Waterford and spent a year there and never worked so hard in my life. Well, there was a working coal mine there and of course I was on first floor. That was admissions and I had a ward full of men. I would come off duty literally black, each time I put my uniform in the sink and my stockings and everything else. The men came right out of the mine and of course they were dirty, filthy dirty, and by the time you washed off the area injured for x-rays, bandages, sutures or whatever, you were a dirty mess, resembling the coal miner himself.

There were certain aspects of nursing that didn't appeal to me. I hated obstetrics. I liked surgery, and medical nursing was OK. Pediatrics was good. If you didn't have to give children needles, you were their best friend in the whole world but once you went after them with an injection, they sort of looked at you suspiciously, with fear. Otherwise you could not get through the door fast enough and their little arms were around you. You were a surrogate mother to them while they were there, so I enjoyed that. I love kids.

After that I worked a year at the Nova Scotia Hospital in Dartmouth. Two of us tried to get an apartment with no success because we were Black. When I spoke to the superintendent about it, she was not surprised. She said she had one Black nurse graduating at the time, and they could not have graduation exercises at (I think it was) the Lord Nelson. They had to move the graduation to another location. Our mouths literally dropped because while we were going to school, yes other kids called you the "N" word, but you just coped with it. I grew up in Whitney Pier and there was quite a mixture of nationalities. Anyway, the superintendent said she would let us have a double room in residence and we could stay there as long as we wanted. That is how we got accommodations at the Nova Scotia Hospital. I really enjoyed it there.

Then I went to Belmont, Massachusetts to take a postgraduate course in psychiatry, because I liked it. I came back and applied to the Montreal General because I had heard they had a psych unit, actually they had two. It was terrific. I enjoyed two sessions of working at the Montreal General in psychiatry.

I think the greatest joy was when I was away and I met patients outside of the hospital and they were so glad to see me. The heartache involved in all nursing is if you go on with somebody and you lose them; there is nothing you can say to relatives that puts you in their shoes, especially the death of a young person. I think my most memorable accomplishment was working at the correctional centre. It was a challenge and you were on your own except one day a week when a doctor would come in and see a large number of them. You more or less had to evaluate and go ahead with what you thought needed to be done. It was great because you got to use the knowledge you had to assess people. You got inmates that were rude or used foul language and after a while I would say to them: "If you can't speak to me in a respectable manner, I don't have to take that." I would turn on my heels and walk away saying "when you calm down, I will listen." They would send for you again. Not everybody is cut out for that type of work and not everybody can cope with that type of work. I worked alone as the RN in charge of health service. Today the Correctional Centre employs four nurses.

I retired from nursing due to old age. I fractured my ankle. The demands were far beyond what I could cope with. Nursing today has become more academic. They are not getting the practical experience that we had. It will go its circle. Hands-on situations mean the world to people. Once your mom shows you how to make a cake and says "Okay, I'm going to stand right here," you never forget hands-on learning. Not enough time is given to nursing students for actual hospital experience today.

## BETTY (MACLELLAN) DOWE

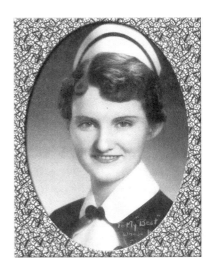

*B*etty *graduated from St. Joseph's Hospital School of Nursing, Glace Bay, in 1957 and began a varied career, primarily in education and administration. Her memories include the aftermath of the No. 26 mine explosion in 1979, the administrative health care changes of her working decades and her experience of joining a national hospital accreditation team. Betty retired in 1994 and has embraced the concept of lifelong learning.*

As you grow older, you remember only the good things. When we were student nurses our lives were very, very controlled because we had to live in residence and we had very strict rules. And we had curfews. We had to be in at ten every night. There was a pond we used to go skating on and the nuns were very strict about wearing slacks, but if you went out with your skates in your hand, it was okay to wear slacks. There were times we went out with our skates in hand and put them under the step. We were given a great deal of responsibility and we seemed to be able to handle it, even at a young age. The big thing was the fellowship we had. I don't know if I can explain how precious that was to all of us. It was really the thing that made nursing education.

Before I was finished, I was offered a job as an instructor in the school of nursing and I took it because I needed to be home. At that time my brother was in medical school and part of my goal was to help support him so that he could finish his education. Then I decided to test my wings and went to work in New York, the big city. I stayed there for six months and got to see everything and decided this is not where I want to be for the rest of my life. I came back and took a postgraduate course in psychiatric nursing. I taught psychiatric nursing to the students here. I taught for thirteen years.

I met my former director of nursing and she asked me if I ever got my degree. I said I couldn't do that, I have two children and she said that was an excuse, not a reason. I found out I could take my science classes here in Sydney. With strong family support, I took the first part of my degree and then decided to go right on to St. FX and finish and I did. Back in the '60s there were not many nursing degrees. I set up the staff education department in Glace Bay and did that for four years and then I became the director of nursing and stayed in that job until the end of my career.

In staff education, I had every department in the hospital and actually one of the biggest challenges of my job was to teach the metric system. We were not using the metric system anywhere in the hospital and the twenty-four hour clock. I had to do it with physicians, nurses, laundry, housekeeping—everybody—and that was a challenge.

I think having gone back and taken my degree later, my children were inspired, because they didn't think there was any way to go but to get a degree. It influenced them, because we did not have to push our kids. They always talked about going to college, because Mom did.

Something that made me the proudest was the way the nurses at our hospital functioned during the 1979 mine explosion at the No. 26 colliery. We received all of the victims, the living and the dead, and the nurses achieved a level of excellence no one could ever have expected. They left their homes to come to work at a moment's notice, got into ambulances and went to Halifax over icy roads. The rest of the nurses that volunteered to come in handled each family dealing with death when the victim was identified. The teamwork, the compassion, the giving of those nurses. It was a very sad day for us in the community and I don't know anyone who did not cry that day.

One of the things that is different today: in the job I was in at that time I was able to keep my finger on the pulse of the whole place and I was visible. The nursing directors were visible and that has changed. It is not that way now. You cannot manage without caring. That is my feeling.

I also was a surveyor of the hospital accreditation, so for eight years I was travelling just a few weeks a year dealing with the hospital but I would be part of a team that would actually go in and survey hospitals. That was right across Canada, so that was a feat for me. I felt that I was learning more than they were learning from me and the hospital accreditation changed from inspection only to consulting and an educational experience.

I retired in 1994. I have not looked back and I have never regretted it. I miss the people and still have a lot of contact with people that I worked with, but I have taken on a life that is just as meaningful and lots of fun. I haven't stopped thinking, learning and doing since I retired.

---

1961: A new wing was added to St. Joseph's Hospital.

---

## JUDY (BURDEN) PRICE

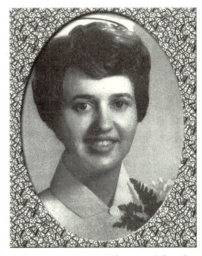

*Judy graduated from Glace Bay General in 1967 and spent most of her nursing career on the surgical units in Glace Bay. She retired in 1999. Judy recalls the challenges and excitement of her career and the close working relationships she enjoyed.*

I love people and I wanted to be a nurse all of my life. I loved the profession for its passion and caring and the self-satisfaction that I got from it. When I graduated and got my RN, I knew I had made the right career choice for me, just being with people, I loved it.

Residence life was a highlight in our career because we became sisters and we lived in residence for three years and solved each other's problems. The first six months of our training was our probation period. We were called "probies." We became part of everybody's family. We still have reunions getting together every year in September in Baddeck or Glace Bay.

When I graduated, I went to work on the surgical floor and worked there my entire nursing career. I enjoyed it very much, working with dressings and drains and the time you spent with the patient when you were doing these procedures was very special. That is what I liked about it. I loved the bedside nursing.

I think the heartache with nursing is that there were so many sad times when you would become so close with a patient and a patient may pass away and you had the closeness with the family. But you could always leave that day knowing that you did your very best. With nursing, I think that there is a spirituality entwined with the profession and it is so important.

We had wonderful working conditions. Everybody helped each other. At that time we were working toward a new building and we had lots of fundraisers. After we moved into the new building we had a surgical floor of course, and it was quite big. There were two wings and the director of nursing thought we should have a few team leaders. So there were about six. You were team leader on your wing and you had the responsibility. It was a challenge, but it worked very well for the floor.

When we worked, the doctors were very well respected and they still are today, but I think the doctor-nurse relationship has changed dramatically. Doctors and nurses have established more of a team relationship. Years ago, doctors were addressed as doctor. When they arrived to make the rounds, the nurses at the desk would immediately stand. Today, the doctor completes rounds alone. The atmosphere is much more relaxed.

I served on many committees over the years. I spent time as a team leader on the surgical, OBS and telemetry units. I helped develop the plans for the surgical pre-admission clinic and thoroughly enjoyed teaching the patients pre- and postoperative and follow-up care.

When you close your eyes and think of a nurse, what do you think of? I think of a white dress uniform, cap and white duty shoes. Times have changed. Nurses today dress for comfort. I think that people in the community, especially the seniors, still look for the white uniforms.

Every day in nursing and modern medicine there are changes and you have to learn to accept those. I know when I was at the new building and we were getting into the year 2000, we were looking at changing the medicine cards and getting meds without cards, now that was a big thing. Ever since we graduated from nursing, we gave meds and had our cards with the name of the patient. This was new and I was on that committee. We worked very hard. We took our floor and talked it over with our colleagues and it was accepted.

I retired in 1999 and things were changing at that time. I see many changes now. We need more nurses on the floor to do the care because that is what the patients are in hospital for. I think the Bachelor of Science in Nursing is an excellent program. I feel the last year should be a full internship allowing the students to get the feel of the hospital routine and working as part of a nursing team. Experience is the best teacher. It is a wonderful career and if I had my day over again I would have chosen nursing as my profession.

---

1971: A report tabled in the Nova Scotia Legislature claimed that the two hospitals in Glace Bay were out of date. At the time, there were 265 beds and a large waiting list.

1978: One hundred citizens of Glace Bay travelled to the capital to protest the government's failure to implement a 1974 election promise made by Gerald Regan to build a new Glace Bay General Hospital.

1979: Premier John Buchanan announced funding for planning for a new hospital in Glace Bay. The phasing out of Glace Bay General Hospital and provincial purchase of St. Joseph's Hospital were announced. St. Joseph's name was changed to Glace Bay Community Hospital.

1981: Construction of the new 125-bed Glace Bay General Hospital began.

# NEW WATERFORD

1913: Two company houses were converted into a 14-bed hospital with accommodations for nursing staff. The hospital was dependent upon miner's subscription dues (known as the check-off) and the general public for financial support. Doctors included Dr. A. W. Miller, Dr. Charles Morrison and Dr. MacLeod. The first surgeon in charge was Dr. R. J. Hartigan. The first matron was Miss Margaret MacDonald, RN. Nurses included Christine MacDonald, Mae Connors and Kathleen Haggerty.

1917: St. Agnes Hall was used as an isolation hospital for a severe smallpox and influenza epidemic.

1924: A new 45-bed facility opened on Plummer Avenue, modelled after the two hospitals in Glace Bay.

1927: A training school for nurses opened under the direction of Mrs. Ethel MacLean. In 1930, the first two graduates were Ida Palmer and Kathleen Murphy.

## EMMA (MacLEAN) MacDONALD

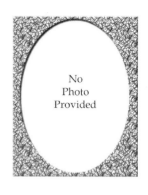

No Photo Provided

*Emma graduated from New Waterford General Hospital School of Nursing in 1940. Like many women of her generation, her nursing career ended when she married in 1947. Emma has retained fond memories of nursing through war time, private duty and life in the operating room where she worked as a supervisor for most of her career. She recalls nursing duties that today's graduates could never imagine.*

I went in 1938. I must have been twenty-two or twenty-three. It had always been in my mind to do it since I was a kid. I loved every bit of it and I would live it over again. It was a three-year course then and we had to be in by 9:45 and lights out were at 10 o'clock. There was one girl who used to get by the window after lights were out and smoke it up and she never got caught. We had a lot of good times. My whole heart and soul was in it and I accomplished it.

When we were students, we gave our patients a bath every morning, we did up the rooms, we did the floors, the windows and had to be ready for inspection. We even had to turn the casters on the bed a certain way and the supervisor would come in and go to each bed in the ward. I was called out of bed one night, I was on night duty, and went over to my room and went to bed and they came knocking at the door and said I was wanted over on second floor by the supervisor. There was a case for the files for the patients and there was a pop bottle in there. I had to get out of bed and take it out and then went back to bed. We cleaned the toilets, we did all that.

When I graduated, I was valedictorian and received two prizes. The supervisor had written out what she thought each one of us would do and she had me going to be a nurse in the army. I had all my papers and she was going to put a good word in for me, but my mother raised such a fuss, it was going to break her heart, so what do you do? You listen to your mother. To this day I regret not being in the services.

I did private duty for a year and then went down to Massachusetts and took a course in operating room. They wanted to keep me down there. It was during the war. The superintendent and the doctors wrote, wanting me to stay, and they would not allow me because they needed their Canadian nurses home. So I came home and I did some more private duty nursing. Then the superintendent of the hospital called me and said she had a private suite case for me if I was interested. It was down at the marine hospital. This patient had spinal meningitis and it was contagious. So there I was with an unconscious patient. I was there for five mornings, dayshifts and the fifth morning I went there the place was empty. The nurse who was on night duty could have called to tell me he had died during the night. To this day, I regret not getting the address of the young boy and his name on his suitcase and it always stayed with me. I would have written to his parents to let them know. It still bothers me.

I was all over the island doing private duty work. We landed at this farm house and the woman had pneumonia and the baby had pneumonia. Her husband worked out on the farm. I was there for about a month and a half. I had a pot under the bed if I had to use it or go outside. There was a stove up in the hall and I would keep that stove going all night. I did the washing, I looked after the two patients, I did the baking, cooking, I was a glorified housekeeper, that is what we were. We were expected to do that. I think I was making $10 for a 24-hour duty. Another time, they asked me if I would go up to Orangedale so I took the morning train and this distinguished man met me at the station and drove me up to what looked like a mansion. I did not know what I was getting myself into. I went in and upstairs there was a little old lady with a big smile who looked like a china doll. I told her who I was and he said: "All I want you to do is stay with her and that is all." He did all the cooking, all the cleaning, everything, and I was there for two months.

I was supervisor of the operating room for seven years and loved it. I don't know what doctors will do without the nurses. When you come right down to it, the doctors have it made. When I was working in the OR, they would have an operation and all they had to do is come in and scrub. Everything was there, the instruments were there, do their job and that was it, leave everything for the nurses to clean up.

Every Christmas, I was Santa Claus. I would have the name of every patient, the families were told Santa was coming and they would leave gifts for whoever was in. I would go around and give them the gifts. Not one patient knew who I was.

I retired in 1947, that was a few years ago. I got married and I wanted to keep working, but my husband did not want me to work and said: "If I can't make enough money for the two of us, there is no sense in us getting married." That is the way he looked at it. I don't think I ever saw anyone pregnant on staff.

It has to be in you and it is not for everybody. I have seen some of the girls just wanting to have the RN behind their name or something and there were a lot of them that should not have been in it; their heart was not in it.

## SISTER BARBARA MULDOON
As told by her brother, Harry Muldoon

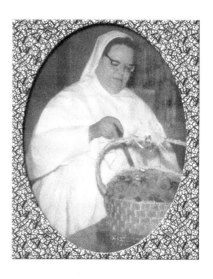

*B*arbara Muldoon graduated from *New Waterford General in 1941. In 1942, she joined the Sisters of St. Martha. Sister Barbara completed a BA at St. FX in 1948 and served in a variety of administrative roles locally and in the U.S. She opened the first school of nursing at the new St. Rita Hospital in 1954. Her brother Harry recalls her tough reputation and the admiration and respect she earned.*

Sister Barbara (Sarah is her right name) went into training in 1938 and graduated in 1941. She joined the Sisters of St. Martha in Antigonish and went on to train with them in the hospital there. She was sent out into the field and went to St. Joseph's in Glace Bay where she worked in a supervisory capacity until the new St. Rita's Hospital was built.

She taught my sister-in-law and my sister. She was tough, real tough. My sister attempted to quit a couple of times. I'd see her coming home and she'd be in tears talking to my mother, saying she wouldn't go back there anymore. Barbara couldn't be lenient on her own kid sister so she had to put the nail to her. Where the students stayed, some of the windows were almost at ground level, easy to go in and out of, you know, and the girls used to skip out. Now, she was in charge of looking after these people and she would have to deal with the parents if anything ever happened. She had ground rules. Anyhow, she knew some of the girls were getting out at night and coming back in without them thinking that she knew about it. So this one particular night she sat by the window in the darkness and they went and started coming back in after 11 o'clock. That would be late by her standards. One of them tripped and made a bit of noise. The other said: "Shh. Don't make too much noise. You're going to wake up Sister Barbara." Sister Barbara put the light on: "Don't worry about me. Sister Barbara is awake."

Sometime in the 1950s she got a request from a cardinal in Massachusetts to come because there was some hospital in trouble there. Within a couple of years they put the hospital back on its feet, her and a couple of sisters from the Marthas. They got it fully accredited. She came back to Antigonish for further studies at St. FX. She got an associated professorship there and she was one of the first to launch the four-year program for nurses. They opened a new hospital in New Waterford, closed down the old General. She went down there supervising. She was there for three or four years and then she was called to Bethany in Antigonish.

In the interim, she started to travel and spent a year in Scotland and England. She toured most of Europe and spent quite a long time in Ireland. She travelled to different parts of the world in her capacity as a nursing instructor. She was over there as an observer to see how European nurses conducted their business. She picked up the nickname "The Flying Nun." That went on for quite a few years until she was called back again to Antigonish. She stayed there until she retired. She retired in 1998 because she had a serious heart attack. They took her to Halifax and did surgery. She never fully recovered and she died in 2000.

She was a firm believer in education, and health issues she was strong on too. You know, supporting the Canadian health system and improving it. She led a commission here in Nova Scotia studying the practice of health in the province. She was also president of the Registered Nurses Association of Nova Scotia and she was on the International Board of Nurses. She had a very active life.

I've seen all kinds of written testimonials to her through the years. At her funeral, in Antigonish, I met more of her former students. They were all different ages. Literally hundreds of them were there that day and the church was full of nurses. They'd say: "If it hadn't been for Sister Barbara, I wouldn't be here today."

## IRENE (HERVE) MACMILLAN

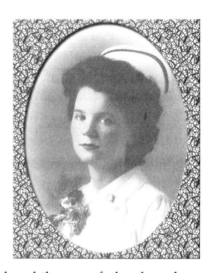

*Irene graduated from New Waterford General in 1946 and began a long career in that community. She worked in a doctor's office, did private duty and worked in administration for more than forty years, retiring as Director of Nursing in 1990. Irene recalls the major changes she witnessed in a half-century of health care and the joys and heartaches of her nursing roles.*

I probably became a nurse because my sister also trained at the Hospital and then my father heard about girls in training there doing so well. The first year I was in training my name was called for being the best student. We worked the whole month without a day off and also did training in class when you were not on the floors. It was $8 a month wages the first year, $10 the second year and $12 the last year.

When I graduated, I led my class. After training at the New Waterford Hospital, I felt like I could take on anything because we were so well trained. I worked as a nurse in a doctor's office for eighteen months. At that time, I was getting married and in those days when you got married, you didn't have a job. I did private duty at night in the hospitals. I received $5 for an eight-hour duty and $7.50 for twelve hours. I had two sons, one in 1950 and the other in 1951. People had to hire their own private nurses because the government and the medical plan and the hospital insurance never covered anything. Patients were charged for everything, including Aspirins. They practically would go bankrupt if they got sick.

In 1952, I got a job evening and night supervising. I was in charge of all the student nurses and the one RN in the building. I kept that up until I got pregnant again in 1956. Then you didn't get any unemployment insurance and you had to quit your job. A year later a supervisor was leaving and I got the job. In 1963, the New Waterford General Hospital closed and we moved into the new hospital and then I had to be rehired once again because the Sisters of St. Martha were going to administer the hospital. They hired me as night supervisor and I kept on with that until 1974, when I went into in-service education for five years.

In 1978, I took a position as Director of Nursing for a year. This grew into another year and so on until I was ready to retire; in all, thirteen years. So when I retired I was the director of nursing and I liked working with the sisters as they treated me very well. This was my favourite position as I was able to help people. I worked until the day I turned sixty-five.

To me, being a nurse meant being there in the time of death, to be the last person sometimes to hold their hand and then you were the first one there at the beginning of life. It was a real privilege. In the early days, people were looked after at home for the simple reason that if they went to hospital, it would cost a clear fortune. In those days, the miners paid into the hospital so the miners got a better rate. Their drugs were not paid for. We had that many babies in the wards that we sometimes would have to take the drawers out of the dressers and then put a pillow and blanket in them with the baby until a bed freed up. If you were in the newborn nursery, you not only had all the babies to look after, bathing and feeding, you also had to make up all those formulas. You also had to wet mop the floor.

In 1965, I went to further my education. I took the nursing unit administration course. When I took over as Director of Nursing I felt I should have a little more education so I applied to take a health care organization and management course. It was a two-year home study course. Patients used to be always glad to see me. I used to love making rounds instead of sitting in the office. My staff trusted me and they knew that if they told me something,

I wouldn't tell anyone or use it against them. You never broke confidentiality. My husband used to ask me how so and so is and I would tell him that I didn't know.

Uniforms are very important to me. If a patient can see a black band on the cap then they know she is a nurse and if they have some problem they wanted to discuss, they could talk to her. It is so important for people to be able to identify who you are and we have lost that. If you have a little badge on your uniform, no one can see that. Half the time they don't even wear one or it has slipped over and you cannot read it. You don't know who is who. I don't mean that one is not as important as the other, but the nurse has a role that someone else cannot fill. I went in with my husband a while ago and I didn't know who was who, unless they had a scope around their neck.

Now the hospitals rely on LPNs more because every nurse that comes out has to have four years university. Some people would be excellent nurses but they cannot afford to go to university. There were no male nurses throughout my training and most of my career. Coming on the 1990s, there were a few male nurses on the scene. We were glad to see them.

## ELEANOR (MORRISON) BURKE

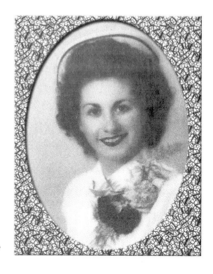

*Eleanor graduated in 1946 and worked most of her career at New Waterford General and later as an occupational health nurse at the Cape Breton Development Corporation (Devco). She remembers the pleasure and hardships of her early nursing years and the unique role of nurses in the coal industry. Life threw Eleanor a curveball when she was widowed with three young children. She supported her family through her profession although she had hoped to stay home with them. Back injury forced her retirement in 1987 but Eleanor's love of nursing remains.*

It was quite a transition for a young girl coming from high school to having the responsibility of looking after people. We were really thrown right into things. I can remember my first evening on duty and this nurse who was a year my senior. I had come into the diet kitchen and I had to sit down, as my feet were killing me. The new shoes and it was the first time. She said: "You'll get used to it, you'll get over it. Have a little rest and then back at it and break those shoes in."

The residence was where I lived and the other girls were like my family. We had to be in at 9:45 and lights out at 10 o'clock, which was impossible. The evening supervisor was very strict and if she wasn't busy, she would be around checking to make sure the lights were out. Things were done right. My roommate would be on back shift trying to sleep during the day and there would be me doing a day shift coming off the shift and she would be trying to get some more sleep before going back in. They didn't have that part planned out well, the sleeping arrangements.

In those days, we did a lot of things that housekeeping does today; like getting the dry mop and mopping all the woollies under the beds, getting the wards ready for the visitors coming in at 7 p.m. In the evenings, when visiting hours were at seven, if you had the lunch for the evening, you went down to the big main kitchen with this huge coal stove and you made the toast over the hot coals and the tea and you had it ready for eight when the visitors left. In the meantime, you had to catch up on the chores that you had left that you were supposed to be doing. If you were on the 11 p.m. shift, you took turns doing the dinners for the whole month and you would come over at ten. Then we didn't have electrical refrigeration, it was ice above this big walk-in freezer and the water would be dripping down the back of your neck. When the cook got the dinner ready, we would buzz the floors and tell them it was ready and then we went up and minded the whole floor while the nurses went down to have their dinner. We even had to set out a place on the kitchen counter for the fireman.

In the case room, when the doctor would let us deliver a baby, that was quite a thrill. I will never forget the first birth I saw. You feel like you are going to faint the first time you see it because it is so ... but then you get used to it.

I never planned on working when I had my children, but my husband died when my youngest daughter wasn't three months old. He died the day before our ninth anniversary and my oldest girl, who is a pharmacist now, was only four-and-a-half, the other was not even three. So I had to go to work. I had housekeepers, not to clean the house, to look after my children. I worked and found it hard because I would rather be home with them. I supervised at the New Waterford Hospital for several years during the evenings and nights, but then it was getting to be too much for me with my children becoming teenagers and I needed to be home for that. When I went to work, I left my troubles at the door so I could concentrate on my work. And I am glad I went into nursing, it was very rewarding. I loved my nursing career, I really did.

In the olden days, say if we were sitting at our desks trying to get a few notes done and a doctor came by, you had to get up from your seat and stand and doctors were very bossy and demanding (although not all of them). Today, doctors are more relaxed and the nurses can talk to them one-on-one as equals.

Anything that happened in the hospital was a secret. I remember going home and my mother asking me if there was "anyone in the hospital I know." I told her I didn't want to be disrespectful, but you are never to ask me because I can never tell you anything that happens within the hospital. She never, ever did. Sometimes a patient will tell you things and I will never reveal anything someone has told you. The patients really trusted you. In the olden days, the ladies used to have the really long hair and wear it up in braids and if you had a patient in a few weeks, and in those days people were in hospital longer, so we had to wash their hair when they were bedridden patients.

With Devco, I was occupational health nurse. We had an office and a treatment room which was fully equipped like the out-patient room at the hospital. Granted, we didn't have the sophisticated resuscitation equipment they had there. We took training in occupational health and how we were to treat the injured. When there was a mine accident, we were called but we didn't have to go underground because we had boys underground, trained technicians. They would phone us from underground to give us the nature of the injury and we would call the hospital to tell them this would be a case we would be bringing up. We would get the ambulance and take them over to the slope that the miners would be coming up from and bring them to the surface and accompany them to the hospital. We would bring them over to our treatment room because most of the time they would be black with dust and they would be cleaned because it wouldn't be nice to bring them to the hospital like that. The men minded that themselves.

Shortly after working at Devco we got together and designed a uniform which included a white collar which was detachable and could be washed. It had a blue tunic top and pants as they were more suitable for bending. After that, any type of blue would be fine. We wore our caps for a while but they would get dirty so quick there. After a while we started wearing lab coats as well.

## LAURA (WATTS) MACKINNON

*Laura graduated from Sydney City Hospital School of Nursing in 1952 and began her career in the medical and surgical units there. She soon became a supervisor and later moved into administration at the New Waterford Hospital. In 1980, Laura began a Bachelor of Administration in health sciences program. Health issues forced her to retire in 1989. She*

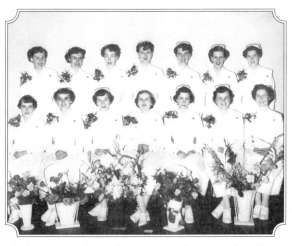

Sydney City, class of 1952. Seated: Iris Mader, Kay Swatko, Marie Jewell, Joan Davison, Mary Kusniak, Shirley Robson, Laura (Watts) MacKinnon. Standing: Mabel Graves, Ann MacLennan, Florence MacIvor, Eleanor Mader, Monica Moffatt, Kay Lamond, Josephine Cruickshank.

*vividly recalls her life in training, the early years of her nursing career and the contrast with the field today.*

I really always wanted to be a nurse. I think it was the idea of being able to help. It wasn't for money because when I first started I was making $24 a week.

The friendships I made in residence were absolutely fabulous. There were only four of us that went in February and today we are still very good friends. I think residence life was the best part. The training was great but it was hard, long hours and very strict. You had to be in every night at 10:15 with lights out at 10:30. There was no fooling around. I think we had a lot put on us when we were so young, but when we were finished we could take responsibility because we were used to doing it. You were just thrown in and that was it. I led my class when I graduated.

After graduation, I went to the third floor at the City Hospital, private rooms with medical and surgical patients combined. The work also involved looking after the central supply room. I would say we had the basic equipment. We had to do our own sterilizing of our syringes. The beds were the old crank style. We also did things like mustard plasters.

As a nurse, my role was as a caregiver and to ensure that the patient was as comfortable as possible and to help the doctor care for the patient. You were also an advocate for the patient.

A memorable accomplishment was being made supervisor the first year after receiving my RN. As a supervisor you were a director, coordinator of different jobs. At the New Waterford Hospital you were also responsible for the plant. If something went wrong, like a fire or power loss, you had to notify the fire station or power company. One night we had a bomb scare. Also, you were a mediator if there was a squabble.

I worked until I had my first child in 1957 and then I didn't go back until 1961. I worked from then on. In New Waterford, things picked up when we moved to the new building. There were some electric beds. There were a lot of time savers and a lot of disposables that we had never seen. I was head nurse of maternity in New Waterford for a couple of years. I went on to be night supervisor. In 1980, I decided to do a Bachelor of Administration in Health Services. I did this by correspondence.

I never saw a male nurse when I was younger. I first saw them as orderlies, then Certified Nursing Assistants. Male nurses have only come about in the past twenty years. I think it is marvelous. There are still a lot of people who find it hard to accept a male. Women are alone with a male doctor and nobody thinks the difference. Male nurses are the greatest thing and we should have had them many years ago.

## CLAIRE (ROACH) TIMMONS

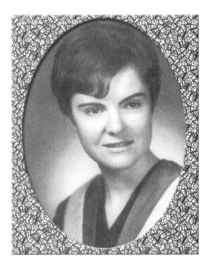

*Claire graduated from the Bachelor of Science in Nursing program at St. Francis Xavier University in 1970. She began her career in her hometown of New Waterford, where she worked first as a staff nurse on a surgical floor and then teaching. Claire also taught at St. Rita School of Nursing, worked as director of nursing in a nursing home and spent nine years in psychiatry. She retired as director of nursing at the hospital in New Waterford in 1997, but returned to nursing several years later and still enjoys her career part-time.*

I loved the hospital atmosphere. My dad had not been well through my growing-up years and I guess I learned to be part of his caregiving and I just wanted to be a caregiver. I was a member of the third class to go through the four-year program at St. FX. Actually, there were only two of us who ended up graduating in the class. There were only four of us to begin with. We developed a close relationship. The combination of the college and nursing atmosphere was nice. We did stay in residence at St. Martha's for awhile so you saw both sides of the fence. It was a little bit of a challenge at St. Martha's because the three-year students were there and when we came on the floor as St. FX students, there were some barbs thrown at us. We were not going to be real nurses, we were just going to be the nurses behind the desk, which was so far from the truth. In those years, we received a lot of clinical experience, a lot more than they are doing now. For some reason, people tended to shy away a little bit, the stereotypes. Getting my degree made it easier to get a teaching job and helped with each position I held.

After graduation, I was working on a surgical floor at the New Waterford Hospital and it was very threatening at first. I had tremendous help from my co-workers and they were extremely supportive as was the head nurse. From there I went into the school for nursing assistants at New Waterford Hospital and taught there for two years. I transferred into St. Rita School of Nursing and I taught there for two years. My second child came along and I stayed home for ten months. Then I became director of nursing at Maple Hill Manor. I think geriatrics was my favourite. It was the most fulfilling.

One of the things that stands out in my mind happened at Maple Hill Manor. Our group of personal care workers did one of the first tests in the province. I guided them through because I was the instructor as well as the director. A lot of people in the course had not been in school or studied for many years. It was a very threatening thing for them, but they were doing the work anyway and you just had to encourage them and give them the confidence to put it down on paper. It was a fourteen-week course. We had lots of fun doing it together and when they all passed, they were so proud of themselves and I was so proud to be a part of that program.

I was somewhat fortunate that I did very little shift work so I didn't have that tug of war that many of the nurses had. That made a big difference raising a family, organizing your home life. So it was very easy for me to talk about the joys of nursing when I did not have to worry about babysitters, shift work, weekends.

I was at Maple Hill Manor for eight years and then I went to psychiatry and worked in the day hospital program at the Cape Breton Hospital for nine years. I transferred out to New Waterford for a year in the mental health clinic. In all my years of nursing, working with staff, as a co-worker and as a teacher, administrator, I had a lot of joy. Certainly, working with the patients, the clients in psychiatry and to see them improve and get on with their lives was joyful.

When I think of the stress in nursing, I think of budget cuts and downsizing and I was right in the middle of that at New

Waterford. You felt like you were in a vice grip because you were between the budget and the staff and patients. Nursing was evolving so quickly and there was so much that was expected of nurses and so little time and resources to fulfill that. I took an early retirement package in 1997, as my mom was ill at the time and there were more cutbacks and more amalgamation. After my mom died in 2000, I actually missed the challenge. I went back on a part-time basis for the next four years and officially retired in 2004.

I don't know where nursing is going. They have to find time to be able to think and assess and to carry out their assessments. Nurses in homes for special care practise a lot of autonomy in the sense that this is where the ball stops a lot of the time. They have to do quick assessments and make quick judgements. This set of skills is very important. It is a very challenging career.

1957: New Waterford General Hospital School of Nursing closed because of falling enrolments and a shortage of teaching staff. In 33 years, about 300 nurses graduated.

1961: A new 88-bed facility was built, opening as the New Waterford Consolidated Hospital in 1963. The first training school for nursing assistants in Cape Breton was established the same year.

1964: Fifteen nursing assistants graduated. The school operated until 1987, with a total of 487 graduates.

# SYDNEY

1902: The Dominion Iron and Steel Company established the Brookland Street Hospital for the care of its workers on a site later to become the Sydney City Hospital.

1918: Sisters of St. Martha congregation purchased Commander J. K. L. Toss's residence on King's Road to treat convalescent soldiers. In 1920, a maternity unit opened under the name of Ross Memorial Hospital. In 1924, the nursing school opened and the first nurses graduated in 1927. A large barn on the property was converted into a training school and nurses residence. In 1929, the hospital's name was changed to St. Rita. The school of nursing closed in 1933. (It was reopened in 1953.)

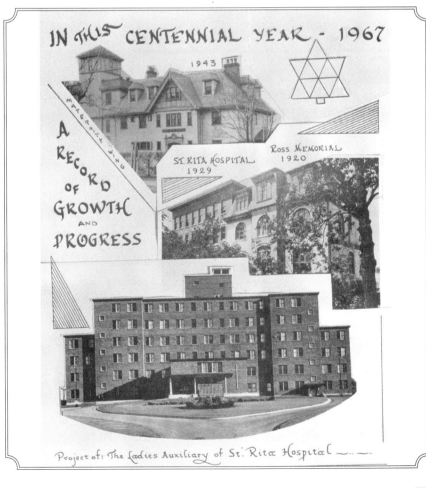

IN THIS CENTENNIAL YEAR - 1967

1943

A RECORD OF GROWTH AND PROGRESS

MATERNITY WING

ST. RITA HOSPITAL 1929

ROSS MEMORIAL 1920

Project of: The Ladies Auxiliary of St. Rita Hospital

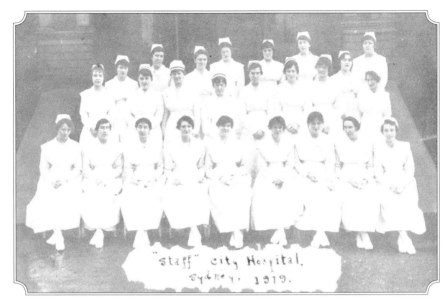

"Staff" Sydney City Hospital, 1919. No other information provided.

## GRACE (WHALEN) BONNAR

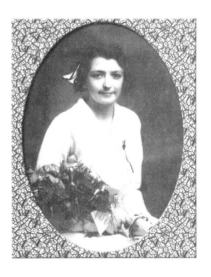

*Grace entered nursing at the age of 16 at Sydney City Hospital School of Nursing and graduated in 1934. Her 25-year career began during the Great Depression and continued through World War II and into modern medical history. She spent her entire nursing career in Cape Breton, working on surgical and geriatric wards and enjoying several stints in the OR. Grace retired for health reasons, but has remained very active, volunteering with health and senior citizens groups.*

I entered training at Sydney City Hospital immediately after high school at the age of sixteen. Consequently, when I graduated, I was too young to write my final exams to get my RN. Then war broke out and I went back and got registered.

Training school was hard. You went to work at 7 a.m., received two hours off in the afternoon and worked until 7 p.m. You worked three shifts then: 7-to-7, 3-to-11 and 11-to-7. Time didn't mean anything. It would be nothing to go until 11 on a 7-to-7 shift. Doctors would come in and dressings needed to be done. You never questioned, you just did what was asked of you.

Of course, in those days you had to make your own uniforms. We started off with six months' probation and at that time you wore your nurse's uniform with black stockings—a plain blue uniform with a white bib and apron. When you finished your six months, then you went into a striped uniform. Third year you had a pink uniform. Now, you don't know who is a nurse and who isn't. They are nice and cheerful in colour, but there should be some distinction. The nurses are losing this distinction. The new degree nurses are bringing with them new uniforms.

I never left Cape Breton to nurse, I nursed here all the time. I started out in male surgical, spent most of my time here until the last two years I worked, when they turned this ward into a geriatrics ward. I went through the OR. I think my favourite place was the OR and I had two stints there.

When I first went into nursing my pay was $5 a day and when I retired it was $10 an hour. Certainly there have been a lot of advancements in medicine with cures and treatments for diseases. I remember when I trained, the contagious disease at that time was tuberculosis, then we came into cancer, then AIDS. It just seems to go through cycles. When my grandfather died in the Victoria General in Halifax, I was sure it was cancer of the stomach, but they didn't know what it was at that time.

I enjoyed and loved nursing and I never went any higher than patient nursing. I never wanted to be a supervisor.

I worked all through the war. I worked thirty-six hours straight when the Newfoundland ship [Caribou] was torpedoed. We had seventy-five private rooms in the hospital and we had to put a partition in each room to put everyone in. We had cots for everyone. It was terrible and to think it was so near our coast.

It only took the probation period for me to become very fond of nursing. I nursed for twenty-five years. When I graduated it was the Great Depression; I was lucky to find work. I think I went home every day with notes in my pocket. It was quite an experience going through all the different stages of medical advancement. I think nurses are born, maybe I am old fashioned. Maybe not so much now. It is a good occupation and there is a lot of work but it is rewarding in many ways. You learn what life is about and how to handle things.

You did many things and the wear and tear on my body is pain from many years as a nurse. When you were finished, you helped others complete their work, in pairs. This way it wasn't a burden and you got to know the different nurses within the hospital. I think this helped a lot. I took early retirement at fifty years old because I developed arthritis of the spine and was off for five weeks for this injury. This was in 1957. After this I went back into work because my husband died and he had worked in the general office for the steel company and at this time employees' pensions died with them. I had worked mostly in surgery and then when I went back after my back injury, I worked in geriatrics.

The thing that struck me most was the idea of going on strike. I realized then there had to be some way for things to improve for us. We worked on and got nothing. We looked around and found out that the garbage collectors were earning more than we got. I think it paid the bills from day to day but you were not able to save anything. The nurses would come to me and say they didn't like how something was going or needed change. I think this kept me young. I was very active. When I retired I became very active with a seniors group. I also belong to the Diabetes Society and look after the foot clinic at the MacGillivray Guest Home. I enjoy it

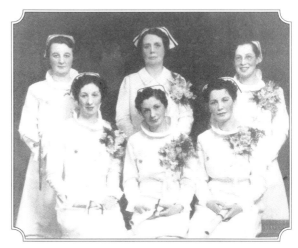

Sydney City Hospital, 1935. Mabel Clark, Helen Campbell, Grace Davis, Jean Price, Glen Morrison

and enjoy meeting people. It keeps you in touch with different things going on.

## MARION (MITCHELL) MACDONALD

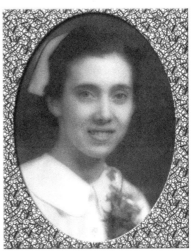

*Marion graduated from Sydney City Hospital in 1937 and worked in the OR. She became a supervisor just a year after graduation. Her nursing career lasted only a few years until her marriage in 1939. Marion has vivid memories of her training days, life during the Great Depression and aspects of nursing that stayed with her over the years.*

My father said: "What do you want to be: a teacher, stenographer or a nurse"? Those were the three choices. I wanted to be a nurse. I would love to have gone to college, but there was no money back then. My school in Stellarton did not have Grade 12 so I was through when I was sixteen and was home three winters. I came to Sydney in 1934 in the depths of the Depression. Sydney was hard stricken and the doctors were scratching for a living, the whole world was in a depression.

A bed in the hospital was $2 but people could not afford it. In the first year of training you would receive $5 a month and out of that was breakage: including books, broken thermometers and all. Some months you would get nothing. When I came down, I did not get home for a year and two months. The junior nurse at night had to get the dinner for all the staff. There was staff over in the TB annex and it was filled. A lot of girls ahead of me in class died of TB. It was rampant. At night you would feed the top dogs first in the diet kitchen on the second floor. They would send soup and the main course up on the lift. Perhaps you would have to cook the potatoes. There was a coal stove in each kitchen. You worked hard and you were never finished on time. They had a maid on each floor but that was not sufficient to do all the work. We did the mopping and the cleaning, the men did the heavy waxing.

You would try to get the floors before the doctors would make the rounds.

The classes were small; there were six in my class. It has been seventy years since I went into training. You were a family. We had dances in the residence and there was a closeness with your classmates. The paid staff was so small, I think the students were how they ran the hospital without great debt. They had the students working, studying and learning. I think the nursing schools were a valuable asset to every community, they were great. My first two weeks in training we went immediately to the floor.

When I finished, I worked in the OR. In 1938, I remember I had the great salary of $60 a month. At the end of that year I got a job as supervisor. I had to arrange the bookings and I think we still had students then. There was a period of about two years. They cut out the nursing school and they reopened it. I loved all my patients and I remember them all. They were so much a part of your life and it was so different than going in and out in a couple of days. You took so much pride in making the patient comfortable. You bathed them, you would at 4 o'clock wash their face and hands and give them a back rub. You knew everyone. It was a different world then.

I retired a week before I was married in 1939. If you were getting married, you were through, everybody was young. No matter what the circumstances of your husband, you didn't work in the hospital.

During World War II, hospital buildings were constructed next to the naval base in Point Edward. The hospital was converted into a suitable institution for the treatment of tuberculosis (TB) and was opened by the Nova Scotia Department of Public Health. In 1949, the matron was Miss Hilda Boutilier. The hospital admitted a total of 252 patients that year.

# ELSIE (DAKAI) PERCY

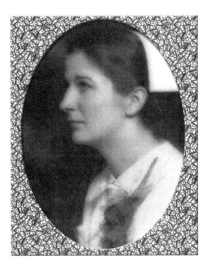

*Elsie graduated from Sydney City Hospital in 1937 and studied public health at McGill University for a year. She began her career with the Victorian Order of Nurses in Montreal, later moving to Dartmouth and back to Cape Breton where she spent most of her career in public health. Elsie retired as a district supervisor in 1978. She recalls working during the war years, changes in public health programs and the pleasures of community nursing.*

I was in training at Sydney City Hospital. I went from 1934 to 1937. We lived in residence. You would have to get up at six o'clock, the housemother would come around and knock. We were on duty from 7 a.m. to 7 p.m. It was a long day, you didn't have time to go anywhere. We were happy anyway, and we were in it together. The senior nurse taught you what to do. You learned to give insulin for injections. You didn't take blood pressures, the doctors took them. You learned on an orange to give an injection.

We didn't get paid anything during the first six months, you were on probation. We were paid very little, but I remember the last year we were paid $5 a month. When you finished training, all you got was $50 a month working at the hospital. After graduation, we were all glad to get a job and proud to be able to wear our uniform and our cap with the black band on it, proud to be through.

Going into public health was what I wanted to do. I wanted to work out in the district, not in a hospital. I took public health at McGill in 1937. The course was a year and then I kept on in Montreal and worked for the VON. I stayed there a year and a half and then went to Dartmouth and worked with the VON until the end of 1940. I came home and worked with public health in Sydney. I worked there from 1941 to 1978; that would be thirty-seven years. I got married in 1942 and at that time you were not allowed to work if you were married. I had to resign. Then they asked me if I would be willing to work because it was war time.

They were kind of short. In a short time I was back to work and worked until 1978.

I worked in Margaree for a year and a half. I came back and worked in the Sydney office. In 1967 to 1968, I went to Dalhousie to take a course in supervision. When I came back, I was supervisor of nurses for the district. I had Cape Breton South which included Sydney, Glace Bay, New Waterford and up as far as Richmond County, Port Hawkesbury and Inverness.

There were no male public health nurses. Male nurses seemed to work in the psychiatric hospitals years ago. We visited all the schools and did the TB testing. There was a lot of TB when I first started to work. We used to do the immunizing in the schools; the doctor did the immunizing but we went with him to organize the children, to get them ready. You would weigh and measure all the children in all the lower grades. Everybody had to be vaccinated for smallpox and we would make sure the kids would be done before starting school.

As a nurse you weren't treating patients, it was more about prevention. We did not do bedside nursing, more promoting good health habits. You just didn't talk about people. We didn't talk about people's conditions to anybody else, it was all confidential. We even had VD clinics in those days. You just did not say anything. It was private.

## ALBERT ORRELL
As told by his son, Dr. Kevin Orrell

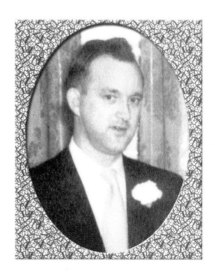

*A*lbert graduated from the Nova Scotia Hospital in 1945 and worked for several years at the Halifax Infirmary. He joined the American Armed Services in 1947 and was stationed at a U.S. naval hospital in New York for two years. Albert returned to Cape Breton and worked for several years at the tuberculosis hospital in Point Edward, at Harbour View Hospital in Sydney Mines and *for a year in Labrador. He later worked at the Cape Breton Hospital and at St. Rita where he was employed at the time of his death in 1982. His son, Dr. Kevin Orrell, recalls his father's early life, his love of nursing and the impact his father's profession had on the Orrell children.*

Albert was born in England in 1922. His mother, an Irish Catholic from Wicklow County, Ireland, served as the local healer and midwife. The family immigrated to Canada when Albert was three. His father had come to Canada to a position as a coal miner in Florence, Cape Breton. In 1931, he died underground in a mine accident. Albert attended school in Sydney Mines and completed high school in Connecticut.

Having always had an interest in medicine, Albert entered the Nova Scotia Hospital three-year diploma program, graduating in 1945. He took a position at the Halifax Infirmary until 1948. During that time, he attempted to enter the Canadian Armed Services. He was declined on medical grounds because of a decrease in hearing in his left ear. He then travelled to the United States and was accepted for service in the American Armed Services. He was stationed in the medical detachment at the U.S. naval hospital in St. Alban's, New York, in the operating room. He received an honourable discharge two years later. He chose to return to Cape Breton and worked for two years at Point Edward Hospital, the tuberculosis hospital of the day. He then went to Harbour View Hospital in Sydney Mines. He also enjoyed a year of travel as an outpost nurse in a remote community in Labrador, returning home to marry, settling in North Sydney and raising five children.

From an early age, I knew my father was unique. Whenever a group was gathered for picnics, camping trips, Boy Scout camps, family reunions or parties, he was always sought for opinions with respect to medical problems. I witnessed him taking care of insect bites and stings, sun stroke, lacerations while swimming, fainting and heart attacks. Many would come to our home to inquire whether they should see their doctor about a specific problem. They would often return to ask for assistance in interpreting what the doctor had advised. He was a leader in the Boy Scout troop at our church and taught many of us first aid during those years.

My father was unique for another reason. He was one of the few male registered nurses in Nova Scotia in the 1960s and 1970s. At the time, I did not appreciate what a rare commodity he was.

There were many tasks in the hospital during those years that were better suited for a male.

He enjoyed the challenge, as well, of working with so many female colleagues.

During the time he was raising his family, Albert was employed at the Cape Breton Hospital and later at St. Rita Hospital. At the time of his premature death from cardiovascular disease in 1982, he was still on staff at St. Rita.

During his early nursing years, Albert was often approached by many of the doctors he worked with to consider entering medical school to become a physician. Although very flattered, he always remained true to the profession he chose. His youngest daughter became a registered nurse. In later years, after his three sons became physicians, he often commented that this was his greatest contribution to the medical profession.

Although many years have gone by since Albert's death, it is not uncommon to hear of people who had contact with him during his years as a nurse working in Cape Breton. Many recall his compassion and kindness and the skill he had as a nurse. He was well known for his medical insight and his common sense. He will always be remembered for the calm way in which he approached urgent or stressful situations. This provided an enormous amount of relief to patients and family members at times of crisis. His children enjoy many stories from former patients or their families. Truly, he is remembered for his compassion and skill and because of his unique position as a male nurse during those years.

## EDNA (FARQUHAR) MACDOUGALL

*E*dna graduated from Jeffrey Hale Hospital, Quebec City in 1941. She served in the navy until the war ended in 1945. Edna returned to Cape Breton and joined the staff of the tuberculosis hospital in Point Edward. After a twenty-year career there, she retired in 1976. Edna recalls the excitement and tragedies of war time, the challenges of long term care and the many personalities she encountered in the health care system.

I thought I'd like to get away from home for awhile so I applied
to three different hospitals and [Jeffrey Hale] was the first one
I heard from. It was a nice hospital, the only English speaking
hospital there at the time. I wanted to see the world. We had lots
of fun and there were a lot of Maritimers in that hospital, too.

There were three supervisors and they were tough. It wasn't
like today. I remember one time when I was getting off early to
come home and catch the train. I was kept on duty later than I
intended to be. I was told I could get off. In those days, they had
a hardwood floor and I can remember I had a tray and I just
finished a prep and there was a big bottle of iodine spilled all
over the newly varnished floor. So I got off early alright. I had
something to remember that supervisor by. She was pretty strict,
but she let me go anyway.

I just stayed a month up there after graduation. Then I came back
to Sydney because my father was sick at the time and my mother
was alone and I had to help her. I did a little bit of private duty in
Sydney at the hospital here and I did a little bit of relief one part
of a summer in the lab at City Hospital.

It was war time then, you know. I wanted to go in the navy so I
applied and got in. And I was in from '43 to the end of the war
in '45. I was stationed in Sydney, Halifax and Newfoundland. We
had a lot of survivors from all the war in the Atlantic here. In the
Gulf of St. Lawrence we had a lot of ships sunk between here and
Newfoundland. So we had a lot of survivors from those ships.

When I got out, I was over here at Point Edward with the
tuberculosis hospital and I was there for twenty years. From
the time it opened to the time it closed. Well, except for about
seven years. I got married and left. But I went back in '59 to the
base. I was superintendent of nurses there for awhile. It was very
interesting. We had lots of experience with the different phases
of tuberculosis and the treatment. It was mostly rest, you know,
in the beginning. Rest because we didn't have the medications
suitable. But they did become available. We had all the latest
medications at that time. That would be about '76 when it closed. I
retired from there.

Becoming superintendent was only by attrition. There were only
several of us and as one retired, the other one took over. I was

supervisor at first. When we had these long-term patients, at Point Edward especially, that was hard. We had patients coming and going when they shouldn't be and we were real policemen sometimes. But that was just because of the fact that they were housed for so long and sick for so long. Most patients are obliging and appreciative.

We did what we thought was right and I think the doctors appreciated it. But I think we treated them with a bit more respect then, probably. I don't know if it's respect, I should say, but it was just a little different. I can remember one doctor we had—he was a nice man, a fine fellow and he loved to come into the hospital. He always liked to have a nurse on either side of him when he was doing his rounds. You had to go with him. But see, they don't do that today. There's nothing as personal. The hospital was smaller and there was a little more personality around.

You see a lot of changes. Changes in the hours of duty for one thing. And the duties that nurses do today rather than what we had. I mean there was a big difference from what they do today— a lot more theory; and we did a lot more menial things, but I'm sure it didn't hurt. I think we did a lot more housekeeping in our first few months of training than the girls have to do today.

I really enjoyed my uniform. I felt great when I had a cap and a bib and an apron. And even after graduation we still wore them, the bib and apron. But it wasn't too long before they changed all that.

Just recently, well in '99, I was out on a ship representing the nursing sisters. They were remembering the sinking of the Caribou. They took us out on the harbour for the afternoon. They laid wreaths out in the Gulf of St. Lawrence in memory of one of the nursing sisters that was lost on the Caribou. It was a touching ceremony.

# Betty Cordeau (Elizabeth)

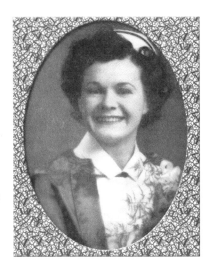

*Betty graduated from Hamilton Hospital School of Nursing, North Sydney, in 1949. She studied public health at the University of Toronto and later completed a Bachelor of Science in Nursing at Mount St. Vincent University. Betty worked as a public health nurse for many years and became the supervisor for Cape Breton Island in 1979. She retired in 1991 after forty years of nursing. Betty shares her memories of the people and places she encountered on the job.*

I always wanted to be a nurse from the time I was a child. My mother always wanted to be a nurse. She met my father and they got married.

I really liked training. We had a lot of fun and we worked hard. We worked all day and had class as soon as we came off duty. We had split shifts so you were working long hours. In certain areas when you were in training, you could be on call for twenty-four hours. We also did lab training and X-ray. It was very strict but we had excellent training. We knew after three years that we were well prepared to work as nursing professionals anywhere on the continent.

I did some private duty nursing after graduation and relief nursing at Harbour View Hospital in Sydney Mines. After attending an orientation in public health nursing, I realized this appealed to me. I went to the University of Toronto to study public health education. When I returned to Cape Breton in 1951, I began working for the Nova Scotia Department of Health in Public Health. My area included all of the Northside and all of Cape Breton County up to Grand Narrows and Piper's Cove. When I first started, tuberculosis was a major health problem. Like all public health nurses, I put great effort into fighting communicable diseases, both with detection and follow-up. We also had regular immunization clinics for diphtheria, whooping cough, polio and tetanus. Later on we added the measles vaccine to our list. We spent a great deal of time in the schools, we did tuberculosis testing and follow-up. Every year the program would be re-evaluated and changed to keep up with improvements and research.

Travelling around Cape Breton presented problems in the 1950s. We had dirt roads. I remember when we first started, we had government cars and they weren't kept in the best of condition. I remember driving on the gravel roads in Barachois. I was crossing the railway track on Barachois Mountain when the car stopped dead. It was stuck right on the railroad track. I jumped out, terrified because I could hear the train. The train stopped in time.

We had to wear a certain length heel and we had to wear Oxfords and a certain length of skirt. Eventually we were allowed to wear slacks, but that was a long time after. We had to wear a cap. If you were caught without your cap on, the penalty was to lose a day's pay. I look back to the strict uniform days and I must admit that I believe in some kind of dress code. Patients in hospitals often complain that they have no way of recognizing a nurse.

I liked working among the general public. We visited all the new babies. I loved this aspect of my work, handling the babies and giving their mothers some advice and answering their questions. I really enjoyed that. We also taught prenatal classes. We used to check the health of all the school children. This included examination of teeth, vision, hearing, spinal column and heads, as well as immunization and tuberculin testing. Every community had its own school and precious little equipment. The nurses had to bring their own pots to boil and sterilize the equipment.

I had so many interesting experiences visiting the schools. I remember a little boy who would come up and talk to me every time I went to his school. The principal would say: "Oh, he's going to be out to see you. He's going to have some reason." She told me he injured his leg. I had him walk for me and asked him what happened. He said: "I don't know. I've just been limping all morning." He was only in Grade 1. I said: "I think we should contact your mother, dear, and she will take you to the doctor." When he was going out, he was limping on the other leg.

I went on to get my Bachelor of Science in Nursing at Mount Saint Vincent University in Halifax. Afterwards, in 1979, I became Supervisor of Public Health for Cape Breton Island. It was a heavy workload and there was no such thing as overtime. It was just understood that you did your work. There were few secretaries and very little help in the office. I took work home at night. More secretaries were hired in later years.

I retired in 1991 because there was an attractive package offered. I had a hard time making up my mind because I loved my work. I decided it was time to do other things. I never felt that nursing was just my job, I devoted my life to it. I do miss it. I miss the interaction with people.

I've seen many changes. My nursing role changed a lot over the years. It's more team work and specialization now. In later years, we worked with speech therapists, dieticians, sanitary inspectors and public health inspectors. We were all interested in prevention.

Although the nursing profession has seen many changes and will continue to see many changes, the essence of nursing will forever remain the same. The primary purpose and focus of the profession has been, is and will always be the health and welfare of the patient.

1941: Sydney City Hospital celebrated its 25th anniversary. In 1949, a fundraising campaign was started to build a new 162-bed hospital on the site of the "old exhibition grounds" overlooking Sydney Harbour. This new St. Rita hospital opened in 1952 at a construction cost of $1.8 million.

1953: The new Sydney City Hospital opened. The $2 million hospital was the site of the new Cape Breton Island Polio Clinic. The school of nursing at St. Rita was reopened. Point Edward Hospital started to train nurse's aides and assistants. In 1956, student nurses from six area hospitals began affiliate training in TB nursing.

## Lynne (Walker) Clarke

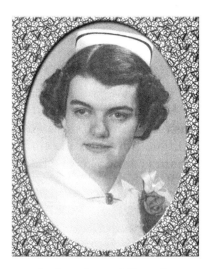

*L*ynn graduated from Sydney City Hospital in 1954 and worked as a psychiatric nurse at the Cape Breton Hospital for most of her career. She witnessed dramatic progress in psychiatric health care, from the days when mental health care was custodial to the modern team approach of active treatment. Lynn spent a number of years in supervisory roles but always preferred direct patient care. She retired in 1993.

Nursing was always one of my desires, to help others. When I graduated from high school, I taught for a year. When I graduated, I wasn't sure if I wanted to be a teacher or a nurse and my experience as a teacher helped me choose to become a nurse. I wanted to be a nurse because I wanted to be part of a team, to help people get their health back. I wanted to help and I felt it was for me as I always had a lot of compassion for the sick.

For the first six months of training, we just studied in class, then wrote our junior RN exams. If we passed them, we were put on the floors for our training. When I was in high school I had to work to receive my grades, but with nursing it just came so easily to me. I felt we received the best training as our instructors were the best and taught us well. During our training, we would do treatments and procedures on the patients with great supervision, which gave us so much confidence. I never felt like I was on my own because we were so well trained. After the three years, we were well equipped to go on to our nursing careers. I made lasting friendships that still exist today. We had lots of laughs. There were only six in our class and the instructors had us under their wings. I trained as a general duty nurse.

Following graduation, I left with a friend to go to Colchester Hospital in Truro for general duty. While there, we worked in every department. We went there for the money. At the Sydney Hospital, they were only paying nurses $95 a month, but at Colchester it was $125.

Later, I returned home due to illness in the family, working at the New Waterford General Hospital. There, you became all too familiar with mining accidents. In 1959, our family moved to Labrador City. With two young children, I could only do relief work.

In 1964, I moved home with my husband and children. I went to the Cape Breton Hospital because I wanted to experience what type of nursing was done in the psychiatry field. When I started, the director of nursing wasn't there a year. She had received the job because she had worked at the Nova Scotia Hospital. At this time there were no supervisors on the floors and the units were being run by untrained attendants. They did all the patient dressings and gave out medications. There were no patient charts and only a few RNs (one per shift) in a hospital with 350 psych patients and another 130 at the adjacent Braemore Home. The RNs went to the pharmacy and organized the patient meds and had the attendants help give them out.

Most disturbing was, in some areas of the hospital, respect for patients was low. I had a burning desire to stay and work toward changes so patients would be given the care and respect needed. Many patients had no contact with their relatives and needed someone to speak on their behalf. Psychiatric drugs were administered with little or no follow up. I had great admiration for some of the attendants who were dedicated and responsible for patient custodial care and daily cleaning and housekeeping duties.

Then the hospital hired a full time psychiatrist who properly prescribed medication. This led to patients improving and eventually being discharged to group homes within the community. Then the hospital hired a physician who began assessing and giving physicals to patients when they were admitted. It was great to see the patients get the help needed. Things at the hospital continuously improved with the addition of a team of psychiatrists, psychologists and MDs on staff. Together with the nurses, team conferences were held discussing each patient's care. It was good to see this finally. It was very challenging and rewarding—quite an experience.

I really didn't like it when we had to come in with street clothes because the uniform created a better relationship with the patient.

The patients told us they preferred us in uniforms. Male nurses were very scarce. We usually looked for a male nurse in the psychiatric setting. When I filled in as director, we started a casual list and took in applications. At that time, there was a shortage of nurses and so we looked into getting some male nurses. In the end of my career we had a few and some CNAs. We had difficult patients and Alzheimer patients, which they were a great help with.

In my last five years, I felt overcome with the office work, which I wasn't trained for and it had become a real problem. I wanted to be with the patient, but you were taken away from that. This meant less and less time to know the progress of the patient. I was most comfortable and got the most pleasure being with a patient and nursing them. I thoroughly enjoyed team nursing and was greatly rewarded by seeing patients develop to their potential.

## CLOTILDA (COWARD) (DOUGLAS) YAKIMCHUK

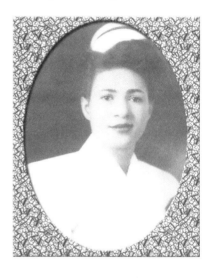

*Clotilda graduated from the Nova Scotia Hospital in 1954 and began an illustrious career in psychiatric nursing and adult education in Nova Scotia and in the Caribbean. She also raised a large family, for many years as a single parent. Clotilda was active in her professional associations and was the first Black woman to head the Registered Nurses Association of Nova Scotia. She retired in 1994 as Director of Education Services at the Cape Breton Regional Hospital. She now hones her skills as a nurse and an educator with groups such as the Retired Nurses Interest Group, the African Nova Scotia Advisory Committee to the Nova Scotia Community College and the Sierra Club of Canada, and is a Member of the Order of Canada.*

I always wanted to be a nurse. I don't know if the uniform or being sick at ten years of age might have helped me focus on nursing. After being turned down by hospitals in Cape Breton, the Nova Scotia Hospital accepted my application. I entered in 1951.

My brother was in pre-med in Halifax at the time. They paid you a small stipend at the end of each month of training. Each year the stipend increased so that is what I used for spending money. That was my attraction to the Nova Scotia Hospital. My brother had the foresight in the '50s to realize that psychiatry and psychiatric nursing was going to be important in terms of health care.

I found that when I finished my training program, I was never out of a job because the Nova Scotia Hospital was known for the calibre of the graduates and the sensitivity that they applied to nursing. I specialized in psychiatric nursing and did postgraduate studies also. I was part of the first postgraduate psychiatric program there and also the first Black person to graduate from the Nova Scotia Hospital School of Nursing. At first, I was afraid for my personal safety. I found that in the Nova Scotia Hospital, you had five or six people that worked on the unit with you, so as far as being left alone as a student, that would have never happened. It was quite a learning experience. I felt we had an advantage because we had exposure to it all and at that time there was very little thought in terms of the connection between physical illness and emotional illness. I think it gave us the edge of looking at the whole person.

When I graduated, I was a prize winner for professional development during my three years. I became a head nurse. It wasn't very long after graduation, I was in charge of the admission unit and the rehabilitation unit. I went to the Caribbean and became director of nursing of a psychiatric hospital in Grenada. In order to be registered, I had to train in midwifery. I had to do thirty deliveries under the supervision of a midwife. In 1957/58, the superintendent of nurses asked me to do some teaching at the Colony Hospital in Grenada. We didn't have any trained staff. I set up basic programs on how to look after a patient, how to take blood pressures, etc. In addition, I established psychiatric nursing programs. We increased our follow-up services, with ex-patients coming in to check on medications, how they were adjusting to home and any great difficulties they might have had. Of course, that follow-up helped in terms of preventing re-admissions. I was seven years at that hospital and in the Caribbean for about twelve years. I was very proud of the training programs I established. When I came back to Canada in 1968, I received a letter of commendation from the Governor of the island.

By that time I had four children. I worked at Sydney City Hospital for a year. You worked your three shifts and having the children small, it became very difficult. I was asked to come for an interview at the Cape Breton Hospital as nursing supervisor. They offered me more money and day shift which was wonderful. In 1973, the government started giving money to hospitals to provide in-service training for staff to maintain and upgrade their skills. So I was the first in-service coordinator at the Cape Breton Hospital. I have always felt, and still do, that I have found my niche in life in the teaching and nursing that I have done. I took an adult education diploma at St. FX and became a visiting instructor at the Nova Scotia Community College, Marconi Campus.

After I had been at the Cape Breton Hospital for a number of years, I started getting involved in our professional association and as a result of that became chair of the Continuing Education Committee for nurses in Cape Breton. When I was elected president of the RN Association of Nova Scotia, it was the first time that a Black person was elected to that position. It was the highlight of my career. The other time would be when I was the first person to receive an honorary diploma from the Nova Scotia Community College.

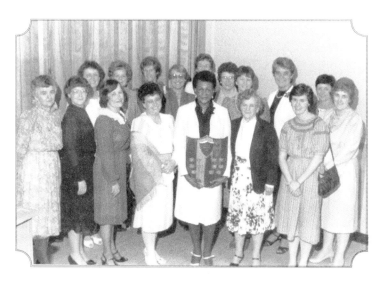

Registered Nurses Association of Nova Scotia, Branch of the Year Award, 1984. Chair, Clotilda Yakimchuk (centre).

I think my biggest accomplishment is raising five children without their father. They were quite small when he died. They are all fairly successful and they all have their own families. They are all productive people. As a single parent, it was never easy. I think I was never without a job. My nursing profession offered me that security. I have been busy since retirement. I do a lot of presentations across Nova Scotia. I have been doing health issues in the Black community for the last number of years.

There is a hierarchy that exists between our nursing colleagues. If you worked in a general hospital, you were always considered the cream of the crop. I was told by one director of nursing that good nurses didn't work in psychiatric facilities and definitely not in nursing homes. I think people are starting to realize the skills, knowledge and expertise required for psychiatry, gerontology; all the skills that encompass the nursing field.

---

1955: The new Cape Breton County Mental Hospital opened in Sydney River, replacing an old facility that was destroyed by fire in 1950.

---

## CAROLINE (GROMICK) PARUCH

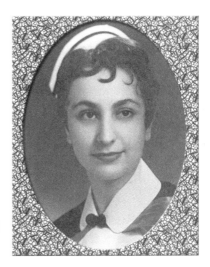

*Caroline graduated from St. Joseph's in 1956. She began a long career in obstetrics with her first position in Sudbury, Ontario. Caroline returned to Cape Breton a few years later and continued working in maternity at St. Rita Hospital. She was involved in patient and staff education toward the end of her career, retiring in 1994. Caroline recalls the challenges of raising a family while working, the changes in healthcare through the decades and her involvement in labour relations.*

I became a nurse because I liked helping people. Nurse's training was not easy and required a great deal of commitment, concentration, responsibility and self-discipline. It was not unusual to work night duty, go to breakfast, sleep in the barracks (at the Sister's residence), wake up and go to class. Our social lives were not too exciting, but it was rewarding working with the patients and learning. We made friends and shared the good and the bad. We laughed and sang a great deal. I believe living in residence made a difference in the camaraderie.

Following graduation, when I obtained my first nursing position in Sudbury, Ontario, I was hired as a delivery room nurse. Obstetrics or mother/baby care became my area of concentration for the greatest part of my nursing career. My first position was a memorable and excellent experience. It forged the way to make maternal and child care my specialty. The staff in the maternity floor/case room were great team members. The administrative staff were obliging, the physicians receptive and the general staff were friendly and cooperative. It was like the League of Nations. I worked with nurses from Ireland, Australia, Portugal, Austria, the Netherlands, Ontario and New Brunswick.

In 1961, my family returned to Cape Breton. I was accepted at St. Rita to do part-time work on the maternity floors. Again I had to resign my position, this time due to a complicated pregnancy of my own. When my daughter was a month old, I accepted a part-time position on the maternity floor and nursery. In 1969, I accepted a full-time position on the maternity floor and case room. It was permanent nights, working with mothers and babies in labour and delivery. To have a healthy outcome was my greatest pleasure. As a staff nurse and education coordinator of the prenatal unit, I enjoyed working with the staff, patients and other health care providers.

Changes were taking place; the hospital adopted the family-centered maternity care concept: rooming in, changes in decor in the nurseries and case rooms. Breast feeding was encouraged. I personally visited all nursing mothers on most days. One of the most memorable accomplishments toward the end of my nursing career was the postpartum education pilot project. St. Rita Hospital was selected by the federal Department of Health to do the testing for the Atlantic provinces. I was appointed to implement the pilot project. It was an excellent program, required a great deal of work, very satisfying and beneficial.

I found it difficult to comprehend that nurses were put in a position where they had to go on strike in order to meet their socio-economic needs and staffing requirements. In the late 1960s and early 1970s I became involved in the St. Rita staff association as a negotiating team member. I continued on the negotiating team for many years. I served as president of the St. Rita local of the Nova Scotia Nurses Union from 1978 to 1980 and first provincial vice-president. Improvements came about, some quicker than others. Gradually, nurse's socio-economic situations improved. It requires stamina, vigilance, hard work, perseverance and solidarity to maintain good working conditions for nurses. Another disappointment to me was the lack of an uproar from nurses of all categories about the closure of the nursing schools on Cape Breton Island.

I went on sick leave in 1993 and retired in 1994. I have not been in the hospital setting for ten years, but I would like to see nurses more politically active. How we live and how we die involves politics. Whether we like it or not, we are involved. Nursing schools need to be brought back, preferably the three-year program—two years plus a one year internship. Nursing degrees can be obtained, but all nurses do not need degrees. There needs to be more input from staff to improve nursing care. Nursing is a worthwhile profession and cannot be treated as a business.

## DR. MARION (ATKINSON) MACINTOSH

*Marion graduated from Glace Bay General in 1957. She went on to Mount Allison University in Sackville, New Brunswick, and worked as a nurse while she studied to become a doctor. Marion graduated from medical school in 1967 and practised for 35 years, retiring in 2003. She recalls the rigours of training, the value of her nursing skills as she moved into medicine and the changes she observed through her decades in health care.*

No Photo Provided

Our first six months we were called probies, it was our probationary period. We were on the floor and we didn't have an apron. The nurses then had uniforms and the full student nurse's uniform consisted of a blue dress on the inside and then a fluffy apron, starched all around with a bib. We had starched collars and cuffs and then a very starchy hat. For the first six months, you didn't have your hat or bib. You got these at capping time, if you passed your probationary period. Your probationary period was very much classroom. You didn't spend a lot of time on the wards until you got your cap. When we were third-year students we could be in charge of an evening shift, but by that time we were fairly experienced. In your intermediate year, you may have been with a senior student. You would have been taught by the seniors and new grads. There weren't teachers on the floors like there is now. The teaching was done by the person you were working with. That was probably a big change that happened eventually. Then it went down to the two-year program. My experience with two-year people, they needed to be in their jobs for that extra year to get the same confidence and experience. They had to pack a lot of classroom study into those two years. They didn't have the same training on the job.

We lived in residence, of course, and we had a lot of fun. We're planning our 50th high school reunion now and a number of the girls are nurses, too. We graduated together and went into nursing, so I have some fond memories of our time there. People from other communities came in from Sydney Mines, Inverness, all over Cape Breton, so you got to meet people from all over. The work day was pretty hectic. The nurses and the students did all the work. Pretty well all the bed baths were done by us and cleaning bed pans, all those things. We would only mop the floors when the cleaning staff weren't around. We did it in the OR though, as I recall. We definitely did it in labour and delivery and that went on for a long time. It was more in the second year that we learned about medication. We didn't get paid a lot. I think we got $12 a month for our first year and maybe $14 in our second.

After graduation, I went directly into pre-med at Mount A. I knew I wanted more. Training kind of whet my appetite for further study. It was very limited, what you could do. You could become a teacher or a public health nurse, or you could do administration, but there were very few other things. I decided to go into medicine. I just wanted to stay closer to the patient. I did nurse while I was studying medicine. I worked in the OR at the

Sackville Memorial Hospital. I basically worked summers and weekends until my fourth year of medicine and we really didn't have our weekends free after that. I worked also at the emergency department at the VG. Then I went down to Dal and I worked obstetrics. My nursing training certainly helped with the patients. My first year in medicine, my partner and I had a patient and my partner actually fainted, just scared of the patient, an old guy from Camp Hill. Three years of experience with patients had been a lot of help. It was a wonderful thing.

I graduated in 1967 and worked in medicine for 35 years. When I became a doctor, if it wasn't going to make any difference, I wouldn't just order a test. I knew how much work that test was to do. I had to have a reason to do a test. The nurses were pretty well responsible for checking lab results and bringing them to the attention of the doctors. The doctor was the higher up and you were the lower down. It's not like that today. Most health care workers are very much a part of the team.

They were pretty specific about ethics and confidentiality in the beginning of our training. I remember I used to have an awful job with my mother. We just lived so close to the hospital and I would go down and she would ask me: "How is so and so. I heard they were in the hospital." To this day, I don't usually talk about anything that happens in the hospital. My husband was always complaining that some of his parishioners were in the hospital. They'd be my patients and I'd forget to tell him about them and of course confidentiality has changed so much. Everything you do now can be tracked.

We had one male nurse in our class. I think he became pretty much a part of our class. But I was one of the few women in medicine when I first went in. The guys probably felt that you were treated normally, but the professors would come in and say "Gentlemen," totally ignoring the women in the class, so he may have felt differently about that.

In the future of nursing, I see difficulties with trying to get people to work shift work. I mean, that's fine to do when you are a young nurse but as you get older, it's harder for people to deal with this night work. Of course you are going to have to pay them equally to all other health care workers. They are having trouble getting people into nursing for that reason but there still seems to be lots of people who want to get into the Licenced Practical Nursing programs. They get pretty good training, too and they do a good job.

## JIM STRUTHERS

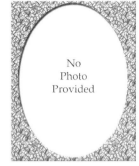

No Photo Provided

*Jim graduated from Glace Bay General in 1957 and completed postgraduate studies in psychiatry, operating room and gerontology. He worked at the Cape Breton Hospital, throughout Canada and in the central African country of Zambia. He completed further studies in theology, was ordained in Christian ministry and is now retired and living in Halifax, Nova Scotia. Jim reflects on the challenges of working in a female dominated profession and on his love of teaching.*

I don't know if it is a philosophical thing or some intuitive sense I was born with, I've always liked the hospital environment and I always wanted to have something to do with sick people. Many critics (including female nurses in the early days) thought I chose nursing because I couldn't become an MD. It was nothing like that, not for me it wasn't anyway.

I really enjoyed the discipline of training. I am just that kind of person, I function better if I am disciplined. I made a lot of good friends. What I didn't like was the long hours. We staffed the hospital working twelve-hour days. I was disappointed that I was not able to take obstetrical nursing. It was not part of the men's training. It proved to be a detriment later on in my career. I lived in residence in the basement. I had my own room and a private bathroom.

Following graduation, I was employed very quickly, along with three female nurses to institute a medication program, a first for the Cape Breton Hospital. Many of the patients at that time were secluded and locked in rooms. We started to give medication. Eventually most were able to enjoy a much better quality of life with the use of major tranquillizers and professional supervision. It was a challenging and rewarding experience.

Personal successes included being asked to teach a personal care workers' course in a nursing home setting. Another major highlight was my mission hospital experience. I studied theology for two years at a church college and was asked to go to Zambia and set up training for nurses there. It was very satisfying and hard work but I enjoyed it. I worked for three years in very adverse conditions, minimal equipment and resources with patients suffering from TB, tropical diseases, severe worm infestations. We implemented a vaccination program for children in nearby African villages. I was privileged to head up a small dispensing clinic.

Back home in Canada, I worked as a nurse/chaplain at a seniors nursing residence and later opened a nursing unit for dementia patients. I conducted nursing assessments for nursing home placements for Northwood in Halifax. My greatest personal satisfaction came from being a mentor to other nurses.

Over the years, I had the impression from several female nurses that I was intruding on their territory and they could not see me as being as qualified as them, but I proved my own worth.

I believe there should be more emphasis on the art of nursing rather than the science of nursing. In my opinion, not everyone has the right mix of personality, stamina, communication skills, compassion and common sense to be a nurse. I would like to see more aggressive recruitment for men in nursing. I have successfully lobbied to have men featured in ads for nursing.

Inter-provincial licensing is an issue of real concern. Most men that choose nursing as a profession are committed to the job. While we are still in a minority, we are here to stay.

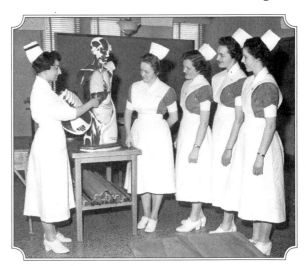

Anatomy class, St. Rita Hospital School of Nursing. No other information provided.

## SHIRLEY MACDONALD

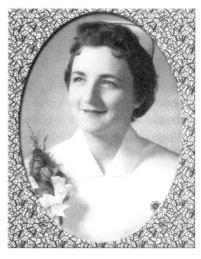

*Shirley graduated from Sydney City Hospital in 1957. She worked at home for a year before marrying and moving to the United States. Shirley has warm memories of her career in maternity and of working with seniors in long term care. She retired in 1997, but still enjoys visiting and helping the elderly.*

I was a little nervous starting out but, overall, it was what I expected. I remember learning to make beds with the tight corners at the bottom in training. We also had to do so at the nurses residence. Even to this day, I still make my bed the same way. I also remember giving my first needle. An elderly gentleman was going to have surgery and the RN took me to his room and asked if he would mind if I gave him his injection. He replied:"No indeed, dear" and took my hand. We couldn't stand around the desk, we had to clean the bed pans, tidy the linen closet. I remember having the towels on the shelves with the folded sides facing the door.

After graduation, I was on the maternity floor for one year. Then I got married and we moved to the U.S. I applied for a job at a hospital and told the administrator I didn't have a Massachusetts registration, that I only had my Nova Scotia registration. She said a nurse from Nova Scotia without is better than one from here with registration. The supervisor on the floor was a graduate from Sydney City Hospital.

I enjoyed bringing the newborn babies to their mothers to be fed and to see families leaving with their babies. In the U.S., I worked at a cancer ward and obstetrics. The cancer patients were only allowed three visitors at a time for the first three days. On the second day, one patient had seven visitors. I had to explain she could only have three. The patient was very angry with me. When I went back to work three days later, she thanked me for telling visitors to leave, because she was so tired.

At the nursing home you almost felt like family because they were often there for a long time. It was difficult having to tell the residents of deaths in their younger families. Especially when it was a child, they would ask why it couldn't have been themselves. It was also hard to watch residents change with Alzheimers and other conditions, so difficult for their families when they would come to visit them.

I would wear my City Hospital cap and the residents would say: "Oh dear, it's nice to see you with your cap on." It would be nice to see nurses go back to white uniforms and caps.

I enjoyed Sunday mornings at the nursing home before dinner. All the residents would be waiting in the lounge and I would play the old church hymns on the piano. They would grasp my hand afterwards. I retired in 1997 for health reasons but, even now, I go to the nursing home along with my husband and sing the church hymns with them. Even if they have Alzheimers, they still remember the hymns and they enjoy it.

> 1958: St. Rita School of Nursing held graduation ceremonies for 18 new nurses and two X-ray technologists. In 1963, Ignatius Hall, a new nursing school and residence, was built.

## ANN (CAMPBELL) D'ANDREA

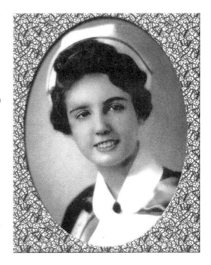

*Ann graduated from St. Elizabeth's Hospital School of Nursing, North Sydney, in 1960 and began a local career that took her from general duty to pediatrics to psychiatric nursing. Ann worked at the Cape Breton Hospital in nursing administration for many years, and ended her career at the Cape Breton Regional Hospital. She retired in 1997 due to illness. Ann recalls the pleasure and pain of patient care and the unique rewards of psychiatric nursing.*

When I finished high school, there weren't too many vocations open to you. You either took the commercial course or you took the academic and if you took the academic, it was either teaching or nursing. If I had my day over again, I would still be a nurse.

I learned a lot about myself in training and about why people behave the way they do. I was an only child and when I came home, I found it very difficult to be by myself again. Living with a bunch of nurses for three years, I missed them like crazy. We all lived in residence and you only got home on Saturday and Sunday for the first six months and after that you were lucky if you got home once a week. The first six months in training, we never got five cents. We got $5 a month after we were "capped" and the last year we got $8. In the last four months we got $20. I tripped one day coming down the stairs, I had gone to CSR to get the tray of thermometers and they all smashed. They took that out of the $5. I lost my cap for two months because my hair was cut too short. I was told my haircut was unprofessional. I also remember being awakened after a back shift to come back to the hospital and empty a wastepaper basket I had forgotten.

I graduated and came and worked at the City. I graduated in September and, by March 21, I was working 3-to-11. It was a huge snow storm and nothing was moving. I was determined to walk home. I was off at eleven and did not get home until two and my parents were all upset because they did not know where I was. I went to bed and around 4 a.m. the man next door called. His wife was in labour. My father had to take me next door, the winds and snow were so bad. We delivered a baby at 6 a.m. The doctor got there just minutes before the actual delivery. He walked in the door behind a snow plow. We took them to St. Rita to the nursery in Filmore's ambulance and it took us a couple of hours to get there. That is something I will never forget.

I worked in pediatrics at St. Rita for four years and the hardest thing was watching children die. I left pediatrics after my first son was born because I found I could not function looking after sick children because I could see my own baby and it was really difficult.

I worked at the Cape Breton Hospital and that is the type of nursing you really have to enjoy to function properly because it is a different type of nursing. There are a lot of ups and downs, but there were a lot of good things, too. You saw people who had been in hospital for years finally being well enough to leave. I spent most of my career there. I went there in 1966 and I ended up there until it closed. I loved psychiatric nursing, I really did. A supervisor had to do a lot more admitting and patient contact. There was more patient contact in the psychiatric setting then because that was part of psychiatric nursing, talking with the patient. That is how you learned what is going on with the patient. There might have been a couple you were scared of but the majority you were not. You wanted to help them because they were shunned by society. I think there were 500 patients when I went there. The hospital was packed and, next door, at the Braemore home there were 60 as well.

I was not a day shift person. I liked evenings and I liked nights because there were not a lot of people around. The doctors were gone. A lot of departments were closed, so nursing became the hospital and it was much easier to work like that. Another thing that was difficult in my career were suicides. They were always hard to handle and I had a few. If you had something traumatic, like a suicide, you would take that home for weeks thinking: "Is there something that I could have done or is there something I didn't do?" It is hard on the families but I guess that is part of life.

There were two male nurses when I went to work at the Cape Breton Hospital but there were quite a few by the time I left there. However, a nurse is a nurse, no difference in my opinion. I had to go back into general nursing for awhile and from there to the Regional until I got sick. When I first went over to the Regional, my feet would be killing me having to walk through the building a couple of times per shift so I had to do what the rest were doing— buy sneakers. Well, I agonized over wearing sneakers, I bought a very expensive pair that looked more like duty shoes but I must say they were a lifesaver.

I have mixed feelings about the nurse practitioner. I think if a nurse wants to be a practitioner, then she should go all the way and be a doctor. Nurses are nurses, it is not medicine. Nursing is a profession all on its own. In my opinion, something has been lost, for both the nurse and the patient, when the nursing students have been removed from the hospital training schools.

## FRANCES (DOUCETTE) MCINTYRE

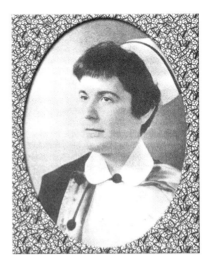

*Frances graduated from St. Elizabeth's Hospital in North Sydney in 1960 and began a local nursing career. She worked in surgery and emergency in area hospitals until 1982, when she began working as a community health nurse in her home community of Membertou and on the other Cape Breton Island First Nations. Frances recalls the cultural challenges she encountered after leaving Membertou and how she applied her new skills during forty years of nursing.*

I wanted something in health care and at that time there was only nursing—so I went into nursing. The only reason I went to North Sydney was because when I was younger, I was shy, and being Native, living on the Membertou Reserve, you never went far. I knew there were two other Native nurses on the Northside who were in their second year so I figured I would not be alone. Being Native we always stuck together. I didn't really have any bad experiences because I am lighter and with the name Doucette, it was considered French, nobody would know that I was native. Half of the time I would just let it be French and could not be bothered to explain who I was. Something about the Northside, they did not know Membertou well anyway.

It was hard work, but it meant money. When we were in training, you only got $5 a month. When I finished, I think I was only making $200 a month but that was a lot of money in the '60s. I still didn't drive, but as soon as I started working I bought a car for my parents. I went to the surgical floor and I worked there for about ten years or more and then I worked as an assistant head nurse. I went to emergency outpatients at St. Rita and from there to Health Canada.

I felt like I was helping people to get better. You would follow them because they would be in a week so you knew their progress. Medical floor, you got to know them better because then you did not have as many nursing homes so people would come to the hospital for a month. I did not like the medical floors because they were like a nursing home. I preferred surgery or emergency and that is where I worked later on.

Being Mi'kmaq, I could speak the language and was able to interpret. Heartaches were when people were dying and you did not know what to do, you just felt for the family. Difficulties were when abusive patients came in and we had to get the police. That is how I went from being shy to assertive. When I worked in outpatients, you were a caregiver, interpreter. Because I came from a different culture, you respected others, whether they were white or other cultures. This made me a better person because I was able to work with other cultures and was able to meet a lot of people.

After working at St. Rita, I started working with community health, with the government. I was able to work in all my native communities and I found I was able to help my people because I worked in Whycocomagh, Chapel Island, Eskasoni and Membertou. I was able to move around, I was able to teach and say: "Hey, you have to be responsible for your own health." We did a lot of programs and prenatal nutrition classes. We did a lot of home care. My clients loved home visits. Maybe you didn't do anything for them, but there are a lot of native elders that are alone and it is to a point now that we don't visit like we used to. When I came home, my work stayed at work and my husband did the same thing. I never talked about anything.

I retired when I turned 60 and figured it is time to retire. I am not registered anymore but in case they need me on the bus, I work for Membertou. They need to do more promoting of nursing in schools, you know, like career days. I think it is the only way it is going to improve because most of the nurses out there are getting older.

## Sister Veronica Matthews

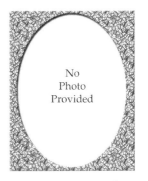

No Photo Provided

*Sr. Veronica graduated from St. Martha's Hospital in Antigonish in 1961 and worked as a pediatric nurse for a decade in Antigonish and Sydney. She continued her education at Dalhousie University, obtaining a BSc in Nursing, majoring in Community Health. Sr. Veronica was on the forefront of home care in eastern Nova Scotia and started a diabetic clinic in her home community of Eskasoni in 1997. She retired in 2002 but remains active in community health.*

My aunt was the first Aboriginal nurse in Canada. She trained in Montreal and she was my father's sister. So there was always an interest in nursing in my family. There were two areas I looked at, that would be nursing and social work. I was born and raised in the Eskasoni community so I'm fluent in the Mi'kmaq language which is a great asset to our own community.

Going back to training, I have some not very good memories because I was the only aboriginal nurse in that class. And most of the people didn't know who I was because of being of mixed race. My father was full-blooded Indian and my mother was half French and they both came from Newfoundland. Some doctors used to make degrading remarks about the Native people, and I was very hurt by it, but never said anything.

I trained at St. Martha's Hospital in Antigonish. We had very good training and, when we finished, we were prepared to run any department in the hospital. My focus when I was in training was pediatrics and I was a pediatric nurse for a number of years at St. Martha's. Then I worked at St. Rita in Sydney for ten years.

The only sad recollection I have of St. Rita Hospital was when the nurses went on strike. I will never forget it. I used to look out the window and see the nurses picketing and I was really torn because I couldn't go on strike, because Sisters of St. Martha owned the hospital at that time. I remember saying to the administrator: "I should be out there." So I was really caught in a bind. That was a very bad experience for me. I couldn't understand the nurses, why they would do that. But looking back now, I understand why all that happened.

The happiest memory I have of my nursing career is that, even at St. Martha's as a very young nurse, some doctor found out that I speak the Mi'kmaq language and they used to call me if there was an Aboriginal person admitted. I would get a call to be the interpreter and to me that was such a great service. When I was at St. Rita, I was constantly called to the emergency to be the interpreter for our people in Eskasoni. Most of these people who couldn't speak the English language didn't really understand it either. They were mostly our elders. I enjoyed doing that. And doctors were very understanding. They knew the importance of knowing what's being done to you and they wouldn't do a procedure unless I came on the scene and explained it to the patient. And I appreciated that. But I didn't realize the service I was providing until I decided to resign from pediatrics and move on.

I went to Dalhousie and did my BSc, in nursing of course, and while I was there I majored in community health nursing. From 1983 I got involved with Martha Home Health Care, that was run by the congregation. Our pilot project became Home Care Nova Scotia. When I switched from hospital nursing to home care, I found home care very demanding and very challenging, but at the same time it was very satisfying and very rewarding, because you were actually taking care of people in their own homes who had nobody to care for them. Community health is very different because you are working at your own pace. It's hard work, you're on your own a lot. You're dealing with the patient and you have to be able to make a decision. For thirteen years, I was a community health nurse; I used to do a lot of home assessments and I really enjoyed that.

I started a diabetic clinic in Eskasoni in 1997 and it is still going. The need was so great and nothing was being done. No one will ever know what we went through getting that clinic off the ground. We had to educate people about diabetes; the prevention and how you care for yourself when you have diabetes. The whole bit. Just the year before that, our community had seven amputations resulting from diabetes.

I can say that confidentiality was not always kept. I used to find when I was doing nursing in a certain area, whatever happened in the department, sometimes you go downtown and you hear it downtown. So I would say that confidentiality was violated many times. Many more than we like to admit.

I retired from nursing in 2002. I travelled for a year to Australia, New Zealand and Hawaii. I was away for a year and I was home about three weeks when I was asked to go back to the clinic three days a week until they got a replacement. That was in September 2003 and I'm still there.

The nursing profession is changing very fast. I think as nurses, and doctors too, we should be more aware of the spiritual needs of the patient. I think what is happening now, we're so dependent on machines and medication that we kind of lose the focus. In that bed is a patient with many spiritual and emotional needs and I think we kind of forget that because we don't have the time. Time is always the factor. Personal contact with the patient is important. Even a touch, if you can't speak to the patient, at least touch them. You know, touch is therapeutic. I really believe that.

## CAROLE RAVANELLO

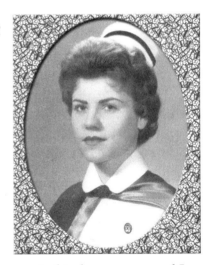

*Carole graduated from St. Rita in 1962 and worked locally for a year before moving to southern California where she nursed in emergency, in the operating room and in a youth health center. She never lost touch with her native island, moving back and forth between Cape Breton and California over three decades. Carole retired in 1994 and began a new career in Cape Breton, operating a bed and breakfast. She recently sold that business.*

I grew up always with the idea of being a nurse. I remember my mother wanted to be a nurse and I think that kind of stuck with me. The first few months in training you do a lot of classroom work, which I liked and excelled in. Then they started sending us to the wards for taking temperatures and blood pressures, feeding patients. It was really a shock to my system and I found out later it is to many young nurses when

SYDNEY

you actually get into the nursing part of it. I remember going into a room with a tray, it was a private room, and the man sitting on the bed had an amputated arm. He was talking to me and the stump was moving around. I went into the utility room and shook all over and said: "I just can't do this." I went to my director of nursing and told her I had to drop out. She told me to go home for a few weeks and think about it. I went back with a different attitude and I made the right decision. By the time we got into our second and definitely our third year, we were put on night duty and you had full responsibility of that ward. By the time we finished our third year, we felt very confident. It was a good career for me and wherever I went, I could get a good job.

I worked for a year at St. Rita before going to southern California with a group of my friends. I worked in the emergency room and I liked that. Then I worked the surgical wards. I worked in the U.S. and came back to Canada on three different occasions, from 1967 to 1968 and from 1975 to 1982, worked at St. Rita as a float person. I took either a three or six-week course in OR technique and worked at the City for a couple of years. I really liked the operating room. It remained my favourite part of nursing and that was where I finished, in the operating room. The drama of it all was so different than bedside nursing. Of course, we didn't have the patient contact, but maybe it was the drama of it.

I went back to California in 1982 and in 1983 I started working for Huntington Beach Hospital. I became a gastro-intestinal lab nurse, working with gastroscopes and exams. I worked doing that for five years and then developed a sensitivity to some of the disinfectants I was using in the scopes. I always had a scratchy throat so I got myself out of there and worked in the same hospital in the recovery room for over a year. Then they had an opening in the operating room. I stayed there until I moved back in 1994. I actually had to give it up. I had three back injuries. Nursing is hard on the back. It got to the point that I was constantly in sciatic discomfort and I was told I had to give up the operating room. It actually made me cry at the time, it was a difficult part in my life. They tried to retrain me. I was in an office and that was okay for a little while.

When I came home for my fall vacation, I purchased a property in Louisbourg and turned it into a bed and breakfast. I started that in

1995. Nursing taught me a lot. I always felt this was a continuation of my nursing but in a happier environment; you were still making people comfortable in a different way.

Personally, at times, I fear for when I am going to have to be cared for. I just hope that the right kind of care and the caring people are going to be there. I think about it more now that I am getting older. What's it going to be like when I need to be in a hospital and need to be cared for, if it continues that they are short of staff and overworked? They can only do so much, they are only human. I must say I am very disappointed in some of the things I have witnessed in recent years, going in as a patient myself. I don't know what you attribute the change to. There was once a lot more intimacy, a lot more personal interest in the patient. You know, you had a closer relationship. We were like one big family and you knew all the staff. Things have really changed a lot. You had longer contact with the patient. The patient stay was longer and you got to know them and their family. These days it is like going through an assembly line, you are just in one door and out. I have been away from bedside nursing for so long, but I can see by observing that it is so different.

## PHYLLIS BALL

*P*hyllis graduated
from Sydney
City Hospital in 1962
and began a thirty-
five-year career that
took her from bedside
care to teaching and
administration in
hospitals from Cape
Breton to Toronto,
Montreal and back
to Nova Scotia. She
embraced lifelong
learning and new
challenges, doing
postgraduate work
in pediatrics and

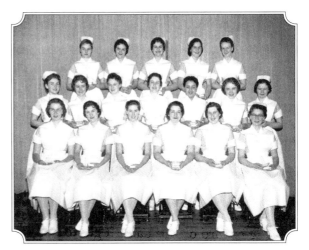

Seated: Gwen Grafton, Sylvia Walton, Murdena Smith, Lorraine Cluett, Lillian Edge, Phyllis Ball. Second row: Joyce Wagner, Shirley MacPherson, Joan Strang, Thelma Timmins, Lydia Brown, Barbara MacQuarrie, Peggy Harvie. Back row: Joan Burns, Grace Banfield, Ellen MacKay, Velma Blakeburn, Iris MacGillivray.

*obtaining her BA. Phyllis first retired in 1994, but was called back
to human resources at the Cape Breton Regional Hospital where she
remained until she retired in 1997. She enjoys new health care roles in her
retirement.*

Nursing was something I always wanted to do and I never
regretted going into training. I have a lot of wonderful memories,
especially the fellowship we had as classmates. We did a lot of
things together. We still keep that fellowship even now, forty-odd
years later.

One of the bad experiences I had was as a probationer. I was
only in training for a couple of months and we had to go over to
do prenatal care and I was sent to a particular unit and assigned
to feed a particular patient. Nobody told me anything about the
patient. When I went into the room she was a very young woman
who had Hodgkin's Disease. This was my first experience for
something like this and it stayed with me a long, long time. I
vowed that I would never do that to anyone else. I would make
sure they knew about the patient before going into the room.

I think some of the joy was the first time I saw the birth of a baby.
My other joy was working with children. I loved working with
them because they could be so sick today and then tomorrow they
are smiling at you. They always smiled at you no matter how sick
they were, they had beautiful smiles on their faces.

When I finished training, five of us moved to Toronto and worked
there. I was on a surgical unit there and my first experience was
a very positive one. Then I went to Halifax and I was on a private
unit there that did medical and surgical. Then a group of us went
to Europe for three months so we didn't have any money when
we came back. Two of us came back to Cape Breton and I worked
in pediatrics. That was in 1965. In 1966, I did postgraduate in
pediatrics at the Montreal Children's Hospital. I was sponsored
and came back to Sydney City Hospital for two years. In 1968, I
was asked to teach pediatrics. I was in the school of nursing until
1974 and then I did in-service education. It was a dual position, it
was in-service plus associate director of nursing. In 1983, I needed
a change. I moved to Halifax and worked at the Grace until 1984.

I have a BA from St. FX. I also have certification in management
(CIM). My personal success would be the way I moved on. I

didn't just stay in one place. I worked in Toronto, I worked again in Halifax and then I came back to Cape Breton and moved back to Halifax until my retirement in 1994. After retirement, I worked part-time in human resources at the Cape Breton Regional Hospital until 1997. I was able to get my degree here in Cape Breton, I taught nursing and went on to be associate director of nursing. Those are some of my personal gains.

I do different things now. I sit on boards. I am one of the coordinators for the Look Good, Feel Better program for cancer patients. I would like to see more bedside nursing. Nurses today try to be at the bedside, but there are so many other things that they have to do. From when I first started and compared with today, the level of care is much more complex.

I think there should be some kind of designation. You cannot tell right now who is a nurse and who is a cleaning person. I think they should have something on their uniform that says RN or LPN, or whatever. I think we have gone too far to the other end of the spectrum.

1965: The province of Nova Scotia took over the Cape Breton Hospital.

1968: Sydney City Hospital opened Urquhart Hall, a new nursing school residence for seventy students. A new cardiac treatment centre opened at Sydney City Hospital in 1972.

1973: The Point Edward Hospital closed due to the decline in TB cases.

1979: The *Cape Breton Post* reported that construction of a new regional hospital would be a decade away.

1980: The Province announced the takeover of Sydney City Hospital. It was described as a "new era of hospital services for Sydney."

1981: The *Cape Breton Post* quoted Nova Scotia's Health minister saying that Sydney needs a regional hospital with facilities similar to the Victoria General Hospital in Halifax. Planning for the new hospital was expected to begin in two years.

1988: The Sisters of St. Martha turned over ownership of St. Rita Hospital to the Province. St. Rita was renamed Sydney Community Health Centre.

1990: Construction of the $90-million regional hospital began at the site on Mira Road near Sydney.

# NORTH SYDNEY / SYDNEY MINES

1911: Hamilton Memorial Hospital School of Nursing opened in North Sydney.

1951: A new wing opened at Harbour View Hospital in Sydney Mines, bringing the total to 102 beds, including a maternity ward.

## NATALIE WILKIE

*Natalie graduated from Hamilton Memorial Hospital School of Nursing in North Sydney in 1952. When Hamilton Hospital closed she moved to the new St. Elizabeth's Hospital nearby. Natalie worked as head nurse on the surgical floor for forty years. She retired in 1993. Natalie has fond memories of her training days and the camaraderie between health care workers that made her career an enjoyable one.*

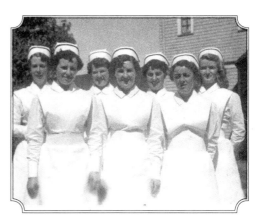

Natalie is in the front row, far right.

I was skiing and I fell down. I had a cartilage removed from my
knee. At the same time, I had an emergency appendectomy. I got
right in with the nurses and I just loved it. I used to watch them.
That's how I decided I wanted to become a nurse. I have happy
memories of training days at the Hamilton Hospital. There were
twelve in our class; I think four went home and eight of us stayed
there. We stayed right in the hospital. The chapel was right below
us in the residence. For the class that lived below us, we used to
pour water down on them through the radiators. We'd torment
them terribly. One night there was someone trying to get in the
front door. We weren't allowed to open the door until the sister
came along. But we opened the door and let the patient in, he was
from Iona. Well, when the sister came, she was so mad she made
us put the patient outside. He rang the doorbell and she let him
in. I will never forget that.

In the case room, there were so many deliveries that you'd take
one to the case room, she wouldn't be ready so we'd have to take
her back and bring another one in. In the meantime, the one in
the room would start having contractions. Oh, we used to have
some wild times. If you worked 3-to-11 you might have gotten to
residence at 2 o'clock in the morning. If you made mistakes, the
sisters called you back and you had to go back over and correct
your mistakes. In the morning, before you went on duty, you had
to have your blue dress on and your bib and apron. You had to
have your scissors, your watch and everything had to be just so.
And if you didn't have everything ready, you weren't allowed
on duty. We had inspection every morning. And you paid for
everything you broke. Sometimes you'd only come home with $5.

We were prepared. We had three years of training. There was
a head nurse working up on the surgical floor and they put
me up there as her assistant. We transferred patients out of
Hamilton Hospital to St. Elizabeth's when we moved down there.
I transferred the last patient. I went on staff and I worked with
a head nurse, then took her place after she left. When we went
down to St. Elizabeth's, we had a course in IV care. There was a
lot of changes. I like the changes and I learned a lot from them. I
wouldn't have made a good head nurse if I hadn't had all those
things. I got along very well with my staff. They were a really good
staff, very attentive with their patients, very caring. We helped
each other, we were like a family, very close.

A personal success was being in charge of the surgical. I was promoted and given the chance to take students. I had a wonderful relationship with the patients. That was my main concern, that the patients were looked after and cared for, that they got the best of care. Heartaches were when you'd have people come in that were very close to me that died. Some of them were really heart breaking. And to see a young child die, it's hard, especially when you get close to people and close to families. It's a hard profession, but I loved it and I would go back to it tomorrow.

I worked the strikes. We'd go in through the back door. It was a hard time, seeing my friends out on strike, walking the picket line. But you had to go in, there was no one to work. It was the management that went to work. One night cops had to come so we could get out. Some of my own staff were very rude to us when we went in in the morning.

I retired in 1993. All the changes started to come. The sisters sold the hospital and the government took over. The paperwork finished me. If I wanted to be a secretary, I would have been a secretary. I wanted to be an RN. I loved being on the floor doing the dressings and going with the doctors. I loved when the patients came back from the OR and we would help them. Working with other nurses, I loved that, but I just had too much paperwork. I couldn't keep up with it.

I didn't think they'd be so short of staff. I thought it would always be the way I left it. We had plenty of staff. You could get on the phone and call people to come in. But now you can't even get people to come in to work. People are working overtime and some of these girls are tired out. I think they should go back to the three-year program. Pay the nurses enough money to keep them here and treat them with respect.

1954: The new St. Elizabeth's Hospital opened in North Sydney, replacing Hamilton Hospital.

## IRENE (STEVENSON) FUNGE

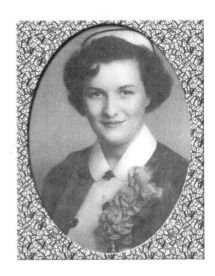

*Irene graduated from St. Elizabeth's Hospital in North Sydney in 1955. She worked briefly in New Waterford, then joined the Royal Canadian Air Force. Irene spent forty years nursing in Canada, Europe and Australia. In 1996, she and her husband returned to Canada to retire. Irene recalls the joys and limitations of military life and her fondness for working with the elderly.*

I am not sure why I chose nursing. In the 1950s, women's career choices were limited. I felt that nursing was what I would be best at. I liked everything in training. I met girls from different parts of Cape Breton. Many are still friends fifty years later. Training was excellent and set me on a path for an interesting life. Without my nursing, I wouldn't have had the opportunity to see as many things as I have. As a student entering, I was naive, but I learned a lot. It was hard work, a lot of discipline and long hours, but rewarding in the end.

I did some private duty after graduation. I worked briefly at New Waterford General Hospital, then I joined the Public Health Department in Sydney. My intent was to attend university to obtain my public health diploma, but there was no placement at the time so I joined the Royal Canadian Air Force. After marriage, as a female officer, release was compulsory, but I continued to work as a civilian nurse for the Department of National Defence, later for the Department of Veteran's Affairs and in other hospitals across Canada, wherever my husband's postings took us. We were fortunate to be assigned to England and France. We lived in Belgium. My career involved all services: medical, surgical, emergency, ICU. Then, in the last ten years, I worked in geriatrics in Australia. There I was the Charge Sister of a retirement village. The village was on sixty acres of land with 300 people living in small homes, along with a 128-unit assisted living hostel and a nursing home. This concept was beneficial to the elderly residents. They were familiar with the staff, the system and the progress from one level to another was not traumatic for them—familiar faces and friends were always close.

All aspects of nursing were interesting but I really liked geriatrics. Getting to know our elderly residents was a joy, they came from all walks of life and had interesting pasts. They had experienced the Great Depression, World War II, they raised families and helped to shape society. Granted, they could be cranky and their care was not always easy. However, they didn't ask for much but a little attention, respect and dignity. When we trained our personal care assistants we tried to emphasize that they treat the elderly as they would like their parents to be treated. No matter what you do in nursing, it is rewarding to see your care turned to good, to see a small improvement in a stroke victim or to see someone leave the hospital healed or improved.

Because I had a husband who was in the military, we moved frequently so my nursing career was often disrupted. I would have to leave my often hard-earned positions and start anew in a new location. For me, it was a personal success to adjust to all these changes, to keep a job and fit into new hospital routines. I enjoyed the challenge of moving and took advantage of opportunities for further education.

I didn't work with any male nurses in Cape Breton, but during my career those I did work with were excellent. Gender was never a problem, we were all part of the same team. I had two male supervisors who were excellent facilitators. When I came back to Canada in 1996, few nursing positions were available and, after forty years, I thought it was time to retire.

Nursing is changing because technology is changing rapidly. Hospital stays are shorter and more care is community-based. Nurses are overworked so there seems to be less time for the personal touch. The degree program is a significant advance. Nurses today are better educated and have a broader base of knowledge than we had.

My hope for the future is that governments will invest more money in our over-extended health care system, increase the number of nursing positions and encourage more nurse practitioners. Yes, I would do it all over again.

## KATHLEEN STEPHENSON

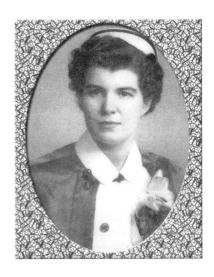

*Kathleen graduated from St. Elizabeth's Hospital in 1955 and began a long career in surgical services at that facility. She also spent several years teaching in the school of nursing and joined the medical division of the Canadian Armed Forces (Reserve) in 1962. Kathleen's additional nursing roles included patient education coordinator and coordinator of quality assurance and risk management. She retired in 1994 and was awarded Honorary Life Membership in the Registered Nurses Association of Nova Scotia for distinguished service.*

I think that from the time I was very, very young, nursing fascinated me. When I graduated, I was too young to go into training so I got a job for three years in the Eaton's order office. It was very interesting and I worked with some older ladies. I learned a lot that helped me as I got along into nursing. I started training at the Hamilton Memorial Hospital in North Sydney in 1952 and then transferred to the new hospital, St. Elizabeth's. I have good memories of the comradeship with our classmates, lots of fun times. We lived very close together, there were only fifteen of us. We were exposed to all the disciplines, but were sent to Halifax for certain disciplines because they felt there was a larger population that would offer more experience. We spent nine months in Halifax for obstetrical training. Then we went to the children's hospital, the TB hospital and the infectious disease hospital.

After graduation, I got a call for surgical services. One of the ladies became ill. I knew the hospital and the routine. This was where I spent most of my career. I was at St. Elizabeth's for thirty-nine years. I spent a couple of years teaching in the school of nursing and I loved it. I think the period of time I was in the school of nursing was the most challenging time that I ever experienced. These were all privately owned hospitals and there was a lot of feeling of ownership. Towns were very supportive. Almost every hospital had a school of nursing. These students

provided services as part of their training so you didn't have
the shortages you have today. You were expected to be able to
transfer from department to department on a moment's notice to
help. Outpatient centres were not established like they are today.
Surgical services also had to look after emergency. You did not get
drop-ins for colds and minor illnesses. Doctors were still making
house calls.

I did postgraduate studies at St. Michael's Hospital in Toronto
in surgical services. I also studied at the [now] Cape Breton
University, mostly courses in sociology and psychology. In 1962,
I became involved in the Reserve component of the Armed
Forces. We did a lot of teaching with the medical assistants. I was
awarded the Armed Forces decoration in 1978.

Another challenge was being an active part of a professional
association. I was on the legislative committee of the RN
association for a period of time and was secretary and vice-
president of the local branches. I was very involved with the
hospital alumni and still am. I was also involved with the Atlantic
Council of Catholic Nurses. I was secretary, president and edited
a newsletter for them. I was a volunteer with the nursing division
of the Emergency Measures Organization and wrote a paper on
the nursing care of mass casualties that was published.

The uniforms were important in the sense that they were
almost a signature, but remember, you were not jumping on
top of stretchers resuscitating people and ambulances were not
equipped like they are today. You didn't have air transport coming
in and landing on the grounds and having to do those types of
things. The white uniform would be very impractical. I think
people have a problem today with identity, you can't tell the
nurse from other workers. I don't know how you would resolve
that, but I don't think the uniform replaces knowledge or
expertise. What older people consider, well there were a lot of
back rubs and serving food that has been taken over by somebody
else. There are hospitals in bigger cities where big firms supply
all the meals, it is a different ball game. So you know, you have to
change with the times.

When I did leave surgical services and became a quality
assurance coordinator, that was another avenue of my life that
was interesting. I was involved in the accreditation process of

the hospital. I was a resource person for the Cape Breton area and provincial hospitals regarding concepts and frameworks for developing quality management programs.

I think the nurse practitioner is a wonderful idea. Some of them are working as private employees of a physician and some in institutions. It is a little slow coming this way because it is a relatively new thing and the centres training them are so far away from us. The ability to get a nursing degree right here on this island is going to make a distinct difference. These people require all this added teaching. There are so many advances in treatment and medications that weren't heard of when we started and I think it is wonderful that this program has come about.

## MARILYN MORRISON FOLEY

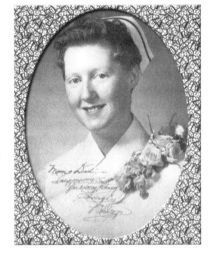

*Marilyn graduated from St. Elizabeth's Hospital in North Sydney in 1956, and began a varied career in OR, medical and psychiatric nursing. She was working in community care in 1992 when her husband's illness led to early retirement. Marilyn has vivid memories of her training days, life on the hospital floors and the continuous learning experiences involved in patient care.*

As a young person, I had no concept of what nurses did. All I saw were women in white caps and uniforms and white shoes. If you went visiting in the hospital, the nurses were finished their work at that time and were doing charting – you didn't see them doing anything. I had the illusion that they didn't do anything. Well, we washed the patients, rubbed their backs and made their beds and helped them get up because the head nurse went with the doctor. On night duty we had to dry mop the floors, clean the bedside tables off. We did a lot on night duty. The utility rooms had to be perfect when we went off duty, the wet wash had to be done and put down the chute. Once you were an RN, you did not have to do that anymore.

I enjoyed the patients. We worked eight hours a day, seven days a week and it was our thrill to get in our uniform and go on duty. I remember one time, when I worked in the case room, one of the ladies called her baby after me and made me feel kind of proud. Getting late passes from residence was a real thrill. We had to be in at ten and of course skating wasn't over until ten—going skating, as if we did not do enough all day running around the hospital.

When I finished, of course, I had plans to go to the Nova Scotia Hospital and take my psychiatric nursing course. In the meantime, I applied for a position at the New Waterford Hospital and I worked there until I went to the Nova Scotia Hospital. I really adored working at the Nova Scotia Hospital. I enjoyed the education, the patients, the staff.

As a student, I loved the OR. I liked the surgical floor more than the medical floor. A surgical patient came in and got well and went home. A medical patient, on the other hand, is in and the condition is usually chronic. It is more of a depressing floor. I liked pediatrics and obstetrics, even though we had hordes of bed wash to do, by hand.

I worked on the maternity floor and one woman had a baby and at first she didn't want to see the baby. I can remember I was flabbergasted, but it made me realize how differently people think. For the mother, it was a passing emotion – mother and baby went home happy and healthy. That was a good learning experience for me. It was always a learning process because you always had different people in with different conditions and situations.

It goes without saying, no remarks about things like this was to leave the floor. Everything was confidential and you would not dare say anything because you might be expelled. That was a no-no.

There was professional dialogue between nurses, head nurses and matrons, and doctors. Yes, I recall standing up when the doctor walked by, but we had been told to by our instructors. Care and treatment was teamwork.

There might have been orderlies or male personal care workers that were able to put a cast on people but they were of the minority, one or two compared to fifteen nurses on a shift. It seemed that when males got into nursing, they did not necessarily stay in the hospital, they went into government jobs or with the drug companies or something like that.

## MARY (CLEARY) MACISSAC

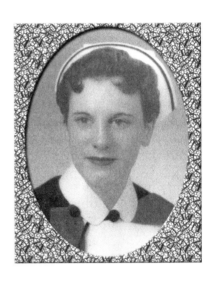

*M*ary graduated from St. Elizabeth's Hospital in 1956 and began a long local career in nursing administration and diabetes education. In 2000, she received an Excellence in Nursing Practice award from the Registered Nurses Association of Nova Scotia for her groundbreaking work in the diabetes community. On her retirement in 2002, Mary received the first Health Care Provider of the Year Award from her employer, the Cape Breton District Health Authority.

I became a nurse because in the 1950s, there were few career options for young women who wished to stay near home and family. Nurse's training at that time started early with hands-on care of patients. I felt I had that something special to offer the patients that I cared for. As these talents unfolded, I knew my decision to become a nurse was the right one for me and I have never wandered in that decision.

I don't recall any bad memories of training days. I recall deep, close friendships that were forged and that have stood the test of time and lasted a lifetime. We prayed together, studied together, laughed together and cried together. We witnessed the miracle of birth, the joy of recovery, the struggle of rehabilitation, the suffering of the ill and injured and the sadness of death. For moments in time, I was an integral part of patients' and families' lives. I feel fortunate to have carried these feelings throughout my career, retaining that wonder at being a healer.

Following graduation, I was a staff member on a medical floor for two years, then in nursing supervision for twenty years. Then twenty years after the start of my career, I specialized in diabetes education. My focus was education and support to people with diabetes, as well as promoting prevention within the community. This was my passion.

I have had an excellent rapport with the physicians I worked with, in some measure due to the small hospital scene. They knew my strengths and weaknesses. Fortunately, I have enjoyed directors of nursing that have been leaders with vision. That also helped me to develop my skill. I value the nurse that works in the field and at my side. I never hesitated to tell them they are valued. The year I retired, I received a special dedication award from the Canadian Diabetes Association.

We are in a period of change in the role of the nurse today. One of the major changes I see is the promotion of leadership the nurse may take. I see a bright future in nursing as nurses take their place of leadership as health care providers.

## TULA (MANCINI) GOUTHRO

*Tula graduated from St. Elizabeth's Hospital in North Sydney in 1956 and began a forty-year career in maternity nursing. She also raised a large family and used her nursing skills outside the hospital. She retired in 1995. Tula's stories illustrate her love of her profession and her keen interest in her specialty.*

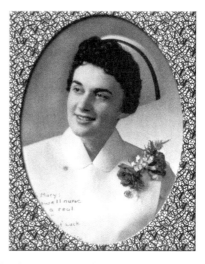

When I was a little girl, I was in hospital with a strep throat and I was so taken with the care that I received from the nursing staff at the hospital, I thought that's what I want to be when I grow up. I was only ten years old at the time. I made lasting friendships in training. We had to work our eight-hour shift duty and then we had to go to classes. We were under the watchful eye of the sisters so we weren't allowed too many privileges. We had to be in by 10 o'clock every night, but it was good training for us. We were only young girls and they were responsible for us. They were more like our parents, really. Every procedure we did, we had to do it three times before we were allowed to do it on our own. They gave us excellent training. We had to report for duty in our bib and aprons. They had the starched collar and our caps had to be perfect. Our shoes had to be polished. If you came on duty with your shoes not quite the way they wanted them, you were sent off the floor and made to polish your shoes. Your laces had to be clean. Your nylons had to be perfect, too.

I got married right away after I graduated and started raising a family. I had seven children, so it was very helpful to me raising my children. If they got sick, I knew what to do. St. Elizabeth's was the only hospital I worked in, really. I did a few shifts at the Harbour View Hospital, which was just in Sydney Mines. It was a small hospital. I did a few private duty cases there. I did work on the medical floor and the surgical floor. I did a bit in outpatients, but my main focus was on maternity. I loved maternity. I've had to deliver about 100 babies on my own. It's much easier to do it in the hospital than at home. We see the parents so happy. I've seen one case where we had triplets. And we had a number of twins.

On maternity, we were usually on a one-to-one basis with the patient. If you were assigned to someone in labour, you followed that patient through to delivery. We worked together and would help one another. If the case room was busy, the postpartem nurse would come and help us. The same with the nursery. I remember one Sunday morning, I was in the nursery and I had twenty-one babies to look after, so I had to call in the troops. We did a lot of helping on the other floors, too, because maternity was not always busy. It comes in phases.

You did a lot of teaching, especially new moms. They had no idea how to make formulas, how to bathe a baby. I even went home with a new mom when I first graduated. I used to go in and make up the baby's formula for the 24-hour period until she was comfortable doing it herself. I used to make these cute little signs for the cribs: "Hi, my name is." If I knew anything about the mother or the father, I'd put it in. The parents would get a charge out of that. Some of them would say they saved that little card and put it in their scrapbook. It caught on and when I wasn't working, they would make one up for the babies.

In obstetrics, a lot of changes were made as far as diagnostic testing went. The ultrasound wasn't heard of when I started. They just had the x-rays. Then fetal monitors came in and prenatal care became much better. You had to be more responsible as far as being educated. You had to learn how to start IVs, learn how to put the patients on the monitors. You had to be retrained.

I retired not too long ago, it was 1995. I was ready to retire then because the twelve-hour shifts were getting a bit much. Nursing is branching out so much now. You need so much education. A lot of the bedside nursing is not like it used to be. They no longer give back rubs to patients. They don't have the time. We used to do a lot of that and comfort our patients that way but we had the time to do that.

## ANN (GOSS) ROBINSON

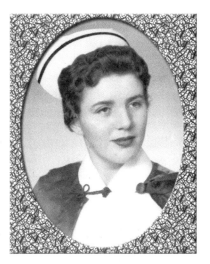

*A*nn *graduated from St. Elizabeth's Hospital in North Sydney in 1957. She worked in obstetrics, surgery and taught in the school of nursing until she went to university in 1969 to study full time, completing a Bachelor of Science in Nursing in 1971. Ann then taught at St. Rita School of Nursing until 1976 when she became Director of Nursing at the Northside General Hospital. In 1982, she assumed additional responsibility for Harbour View Hospital in Sydney Mines. Ann served a variety of roles in the merger of hospitals in industrial Cape Breton in the 1990s and ended her career in administration in Baddeck and Cheticamp. She retired in 1997. Her memories illustrate her love of nursing.*

I look back on my training days with fondness. We received a very good nursing education. After graduation, I continued at St. Elizabeth's. At first I was sort of a generalist, doing obstetrics and I worked in surgery. Then I did some supervision and some clinical teaching in the school of nursing. In 1969, the three-year program finished and I went to university and did my Bachelor of Science in Nursing. I graduated in 1971. Later on I took a distance education course in health care administration through the Canadian Hospital Association. That was another challenge because you had family at home. It was a challenge to maintain your parenting role and your role as a wife. You were a student and you had full-time employment. When I went to university, I did go full-time. The distance education program wasn't available in those days for nurses who wanted to upgrade. We would travel on a Monday morning so we would be in class for 9 a.m. There was another lady that travelled with me, and then we would return on Friday afternoon.

I went to St. Rita Hospital to the school of nursing and I taught there until 1975. I enjoyed the teaching and I learned a lot, I thought. It's interesting and challenging working with the students. I worked in the first-year program. Eventually I realized that I wanted to go back into service. In 1976, I went back to the Northside General, St. Elizabeth's with the name changed. I went back there as Director of Nursing. In the mid-'70s, I served two years as President of the Cape Breton Branch of the Registered Nurses Association of Nova Scotia. In the early '90s, I served two years as a member-at-large and on the board of directors. In '98, I was awarded an Honourary Life Membership to the RNANS.

In 1982, with the opening of the Harbour View Hospital, I became the Assistant Executive Director of Patient Care Services. I was responsible for patient care services in both hospitals. I remained in this position until '95 or '96. We merged all the hospitals. I was involved with the mergers. They needed an interim administrator in Baddeck until the regional boards were ready to have some responsibility for the hospital so I used to travel from North Sydney to Baddeck. I still had responsibilities at the other hospital and I was still involved with the mergers in Sydney. I came to Baddeck two and a half days a week. It was very interesting. There was a certain challenge to it because you were reporting directly to the hospital board. You also worked very closely with the chief of staff and had monthly medical staff meetings. You were responsible for the complete operation of the hospital. The hospital was reasonably new and there were still areas that were being addressed by the architects and the construction people. I would say I had a good relationship with the nurses. Being a nurse, I certainly understood their situation in a small hospital. Then I was asked to go down to Cheticamp two days a week. They were in the process of getting ready to build a new hospital. The hospital was attached to the nursing home. It is a nice operation. I think the two complement each other very much.

When I finished up my assignment in Cheticamp and Baddeck, I retired. That was in 1997. You know when you are ready. Things had begun to change. Nursing has certainly grown in its dimensions, when you think of the different types of nursing we have today: primary care, acute care, home care, nurse practitioners, just to name a few. These people are certainly well equipped, educated to meet the needs of their practice. The bedside nurse is disappearing and that is because of the patient, the illness, the knowledge and the information we have today that we did not have. I nursed for forty-two years and I loved every minute of it. I used to encourage people to have fun and enjoy what they were doing.

Nursing is still a really young profession. It has changed a lot and it will continue to evolve because the health care system is changing so quickly. Nursing will change to meet those needs. It has up to now.

## AMELIA (SYLLIBOY) JESTY

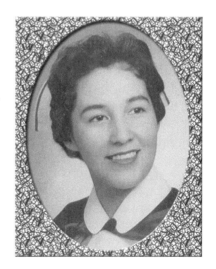

*A*melia graduated from St. Elizabeth's Hospital in North Sydney in 1958. She has had two nursing careers. Amelia worked many years in obstetrics and emergency at Harbour View Hospital in Sydney Mines, retiring in 1987. In 1992, she began a second career as a nursing liaison with First Nations communities. She has worked with First Nations patients at the Cape Breton Regional Hospital for the past seven years. Amelia's fond memories of her early nursing days are mixed with the realities of raising a large family and dealing with prejudice in the health care system.

I am a Mi'kmaq, born and raised in Eskasoni. I guess I chose
nursing because I went to a boarding school for high school
which was in Mabou and the girls were writing applications and
I thought, oh well, I will write an application too. On the First
Nation community we did not have too many role models. We had
a nurse, but she was so isolated from us, and we had nuns and
priests. So what choices did I have? Either be a nun or whatever.
When the girls were saying "I am going into nursing," I thought
okay, I will write out an application—and I got accepted. I entered
training in 1955 and we graduated in 1958 and I received my RN.
We were the first group of students at the new St. Elizabeth's.

Nursing was everything I imagined it to be. Bringing such
pride to my parents and extended family was my greatest thrill.
Graduation was a proud moment. After graduating I joined the
staff at Harbour View Hospital. I think I sort of leaned toward
OBS. OBS was a happy place. I loved the children—babies and
little children. They were the joy. I always liked patients because I
love people.

I do not dwell on those hardships, bad memories or anything like
that. I have many and it was very difficult because I am a First
Nation person and I am sure at times, patients, which I wasn't
aware of, would look and say: "Look who is coming in to fix me up
or to feed me" or whatever. I did get a lot of vibes from that and it
was just a total rejection when I walked in the room, I could feel
it. Grandfather said: "hold your head up high." I think toward the
end I had blocked it out so I did not feel any different than you
or I because I developed such a tough skin. I don't like to go into
details about it because it is not good memories. Discrimination
was rampant and it still is in every institution.

I was at Harbour View for a very long time. I had all my children
when I was working there and they were all born in there. Don't
think a working mother can't raise children. I had seven and
worked right through. I think my children turned out wonderful.
A working mother is a personal success in itself. That is the joy of
life, you have a bunch of children and they were all okay and that
is a satisfaction you don't let go of.

When I started out, we used to make up all the dressings. We had
to do the cleaning up and preparing instruments. We had to do

everything. Not like today, we had to even mop the floors. It was hard work but it was good.

My cap was so important to me because one of the punishments when you did something wrong was to have your cap taken away from you. Getting your cap was a big deal, we had a capping ceremony and that was so important to me. Doctors used to complain when I worked in emergency before I retired and say: "get that thing off your head" because the light would hit it and it would be sideways. I would say: "No, I worked hard for this." I think nurses should wear white uniforms and caps. It is clean and more professional looking.

In 1987, I just got tired of it all. It was getting to be a hassle to go to work, it was no longer a pleasure to go to work. I was in my fifties. I was just tired and all my children left home and now was my time, to pamper me. Everyone said it is wonderful to retire, it is not. I got bored sitting around the house. I returned in 1992, I started with the Native Council of Nova Scotia. I think it was field officer to visit off-reserve natives because I lived off-reserve. I worked for natives in the courts translating and facilitating, helping to retain lawyers, legal aid. I was approached by Corrections Canada. I was dealing with Native offenders. I worked that position for four years.

Today, I am employed by the five First Nations of Cape Breton as a Mi'kmaq interpreter/liaison at the Cape Breton Regional Hospital complex. I assist native clients during their hospital stay by working closely with doctors, nurses and staff. I have been here for seven years and staff are used to seeing me around. Native clients have two barriers to overcome when entering the institution: the English language and hospital terminology. There are a lot of people that will not admit that they don't understand what is being said to them so I will just go back and say: "What did the doctor say?" I have received complaints from patients and I usually get them to write them out and I address the complaints to the right staff. The staff will call me also. I really enjoy it. I hope to continue working with my native people as long as I can, as I see a great need.

## Ann Marie (Day) (Grandy) Steele

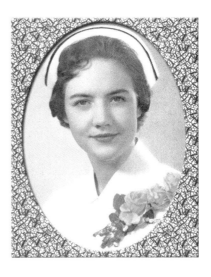

*A*nn Marie graduated from St. Elizabeth's Hospital in North Sydney in 1958 and worked most of her career as head nurse in the ambulatory care/emergency department at that facility. She has fond memories of her training days under the supervision of the Sisters of Charity and of the infancy and growth of emergency and outpatient services in the early days of her career. Ann Marie retired in 1994 after thirty-six years of service. In 2001, she was awarded an honorary life membership in the Registered Nurses Association of Nova Scotia.

From a very young age, nursing was my dream and I was always confident I would succeed. I entered St. Elizabeth Hospital Nursing School in 1955 immediately following my high school graduation. I was seventeen years old.

I entered a three-year program. Following the first six months of classes, we were finally sent to the floors with close supervision, for our hands-on experience. And we got plenty of it. Over the three years we were exposed to medical, surgical, pediatric, maternity and operating room. After a year, we were given a fair bit of responsibility and we accepted it without question. The hospital was run by the Sisters of Charity and there was always a sister supervisor on duty to turn to, or hide from, as the case might be! I feel that we received an excellent education under the guidance of the sisters who sought to teach us compassion, nursing technology, responsibility and a very good work ethic.

We had the opportunity to affiliate at the TB hospital in Point Edward or Halifax for communicable disease training. We also spent three months at the Children's Hospital in Halifax for pediatric nursing and three months at the Halifax Infirmary for additional pediatric and maternity nursing. I enjoyed all three affiliations as meeting students and staff of other hospitals broadened our perspectives. I was the first nurse at St. Elizabeth's to work in the recovery room. I was the senior student assigned there the day it opened in 1958.

The doctors demanded the respect of the young students. If a doctor approached the desk, you immediately stood up and acknowledged their presence. The doctors were very distinguished looking in their two- or three-piece suits. A nurse always made patient rounds with the doctor and wrote his orders as they went along. Today things are much different. It is difficult to tell a doctor or a nurse. Doctors dress very casually and nurses no longer wear a white uniform or a cap. What a shame! In the earlier years, there were very few female doctors so it is nice to see this change.

Following graduation, I continued to work at St. Elizabeth's Hospital. For a short period I was in the operating room. Then I did a two-year term as a nursing arts instructor. I enjoyed the interaction with students, but decided I would like to be more involved with hands-on nursing. In 1961, they were considering opening an outpatient department. Prior to this, all lacerations and emergencies were treated in the operating room, a few emergencies would throw everything into a spin! Since I had some experience, I was asked to set up an outpatient department. At first it was just staffed on day shift. After a number of years and with the expansion of facilities, we were staffed round the clock.

I continued to work in outpatients/emergency for the remainder of my career while keeping up to date by taking courses in continuing education and nursing administration. In the early years, the EKG department was included in outpatients and staff did the EKGs on both outpatients and inpatients. We were also the chemotherapy area and nurses mixed the drugs in the department until we realized how toxic the drugs were without proper ventilation. From 1960 until about 1968, doctors administered general anesthetics in the department for procedures such as teeth extractions, examinations and severe lacerations. I was certainly relieved when that practice changed. I remember that, just like today, we were usually short of staff.

One of my greatest joys was experiencing the birth of a baby for the first time and there was always a heartache when you experienced sudden, unexpected death. In my career, I have found that nurses have more experience dealing with the death of a patient than the doctors. The nurses are the people at the bedside and doctors are rarely there when a death actually takes place.

In 1994, I retired from nursing after working for thirty-six years; thirty-four as head nurse—nursing manager—in ambulatory care/emergency. I can honestly say that nursing was very good to me. There were a few, but not too many, days when I didn't look forward to getting up for work. However, I worked all eight-hour day shifts, no night shifts, which can certainly wear nurses out.

Nursing was everything I dreamed it would be.

## JANE (DeLESKIE) JESSOME

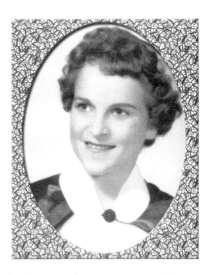

*Jane was born in Whitney Pier and graduated from St. Elizabeth's Hospital in North Sydney in 1961. She stayed at this facility for a long and illustrious career, working first in maternity and later moving into a wide range of management roles that included tremendous community involvement. Jane has continued to serve into her retirement and is especially proud of her work with the blood pressure clinic, the Alzheimer Society and the organ donation program. She established the retired nurses interest group. Her memories summarize the realities of both bedside nursing and health care administration in the last decades of the 20th century.*

When I was young and as a teenager, the sight of blood would make me faint, but I always wanted to be a nurse. I always knew that I wanted to help people. The fact that my mother died when I was six might have had something to do with it because she died at home. In those days, you didn't go to the hospital and I think that might have stayed with me and I wanted to help others in the same situation. I don't have any regrets. I enjoyed nursing. I meet people today and they tell me "how good you made me feel having my first baby, or you were around when my mother died." You realize the impact you had on them. Although you

don't remember it because they were everyday occurrences, to
them you stand out. I think the first time someone died, it is a
shock—you were not used to it. After awhile, you got used to it
and concentrated on comforting the family. In the early days you
would have to wash them after they died, wrap them in a shroud
and take them to the morgue. We did all that.

Immediately following graduation, I did work in pediatrics
because that is where the opening was and then I left to have one
of my children and went back to work in maternity. The maternity
ward was very busy then. There would be 20–25 babies in the
nursery with one RN. Nothing was disposable. We had the old
wringer washers.

When I did write my RNs, I had the second-highest in the
province. I got married and had five children and went back to
work after having every one of them. That was an achievement.
At that time there was no unemployment insurance. Not only
did you resign, you had to resign, you may only get back to work
six months and you would be resigning again because you were
expecting again. You could not work beyond your seventh month,
you had to resign, then you had to reapply. There was lots of work
in those days. You lost your seniority, you lost out on your pension
for those years. It is a lot different from today. I worked a lot of
school events, Christmas Days. One year, I worked back shift and
we had this horrendous storm and I did not get out of the hospital
until after dinner. Needless to say they opened their gifts, their
Dad was always there.

I was a shift supervisor from 1974 to 1989 and I enjoyed that. It
was a challenging and satisfying position. I was in charge of the
whole hospital; went to every crisis situation you could, filled
medications from the pharmacy, called priests and ministers for
the dying or those in bad accidents. I comforted families, started
intravenous, delivered babies. No job description would cover this
position, but it was very rewarding to me.

In 1992, I went to bed utilization officer and also became
responsible for a workload management tool called "GRASP."
That was probably the most dissatisfying part of my whole career.
I would have to go to the nursing units every morning and try
to persuade the physicians to discharge patients who were not
receiving active medical treatment. The ER unit would be calling

because their unit was full of people on stretchers waiting for beds.

I didn't have time in the early years working and having five children too, but as they grew older I did my degree through distance education. Instead of a Bachelor of Nursing, I took a Bachelor in Administration and Health Services which covered a wider range of topics. I did my thesis for my degree on organ donation, public and professional awareness. We came up with the idea of a video on organ donation; it involved students and a lot of staff. I went one step further and got three or four people whose children had died. They came in and told their story. On the other side of the coin, we had people come in who had received an organ and they told their story.

Male nurses, I think we had one in Sydney Mines at that hospital and we had one at the Northside. Today there are quite a few, that stigma is not there. I have a son who is a male registered nurse and he works in ER. I think there are three or four male nurses in ER, just in North Sydney. I had a couple on my staff and they are over in Sydney now. So I think the stigma is no longer there anymore, or if it is, it is very minute.

I retired because I turned 55, but I did give it a lot of thought. I thought I would be here until I was 65 because I really enjoyed it. Coming on the last few years I was not doing one job, but three, four, five jobs, and the stress was taking over and the job satisfaction was going down. The first two years after retiring were hard. I missed not the work, I think I missed the people and I think that is when I started to think more and more about starting the retired nurses group. I started this in February of 1999. The first meeting we had only 33 retired nurses, but today there are more than 133. I believe it proves that we have a unique bond, no matter where we lived or worked.

I think we are missing something today. We have our four-year program which makes great nurses—full of theory, but no hands-on work. They make great teachers, managers, but I think because of the four-year program, hands-on nursing is suffering. We have our LPNs that do a lot and have taken on a lot more responsibilities, but somewhere in there we need something to replace the two-year program. I think one of the biggest complaints today is the bedside nursing, they don't have time to talk anymore and that is a big part of healing. Being able to talk—that is why a lot of retired nurses are such good talkers.

## ETHEL (SQUAREY) CLUETT

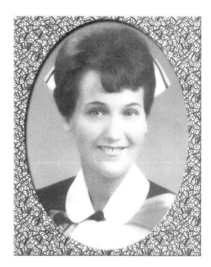

*Ethel graduated from St. Elizabeth's Hospital in North Sydney in 1963. She began her career there and moved to Harbour View Hospital in Sydney Mines where she spent many years in emergency. Ethel later trained and worked as a rehab nurse and retired in 1993 due to illness. She is a life member of the Registered Nurses Association and remains active in her church and her profession.*

I grew up in Port Aux Basques, Newfoundland, and I came to the hospital with an accent, shy and green as grass. I always wanted to go into ministry ... but women didn't do that at that time. The next caring profession was nursing. So I came to Cape Breton because it was closer, it was only eight or nine hours on a boat. If you went to St. John's to a training school, it took two days on a train.

I found it very difficult with the religion—growing up all my life as an Anglican, not ever seeing a Catholic in my life. Everything was very strange to me when I went there and I had to overcome a lot of my problems, or so I thought, with the accent. I learned so much about tolerance. Nursing brought out so much from inside. It gave me a real good self-image. That was the growing and maturing of me. When we graduated, we were sure confident. My mother and father were so proud of what I had done. Mum was coming up in September to see me graduate. Then she had a stroke. That was the only thing about my graduation that I missed—she wasn't there.

After graduation, I was assigned to first floor medical at St. Elizabeth's. I was there for a year and then I came down to Harbour View in Sydney Mines. And that had to be the best place in the world to work. I found it was sort of like a family. You could

really, really care about people. You had a little bit more time.
Not that you weren't rushing around, but you had the people
for a longer time. I liked the fast pace in outpatients, until I got
older. I had nursed for eighteen or nineteen years in outpatients
so I think I had worn myself out. When the old building closed,
everyone went to North Sydney. I was there about four years
and getting older so, when a position came with rehab, I went
to Halifax to get training. It was a different kind of training.
Emergency is so fast and in rehab you have to let other people do
it, the patients. So it was quite a change.

It's like a wheel and everyone has a job and this is what makes
the wheel go round. My pet peeve was dirty shoes and laces.
Nurses coming in in their dirty uniforms. Every time I came off
duty, I brought my laces home and washed them. But now they
wear their shoes to work. We had to take our ordinary shoes off
when we got there and put our nurse's shoes on. I think it's pride
in yourself, too. I think it was the worst thing to take nursing
training out of the hospitals because they had the patient right
there. Something is missing. I think they should be given some
time in a hospital. I know they will say that they do that, but
not enough. Not everybody is going to be an administrator or
director. Somebody's got to do the bedpans, the IVs and the
catheterizations. A lot of things have changed since I left nursing.
I think being a listener is the most important thing because you
can see things you wouldn't if you were in a rush.

I had open heart surgery and to make a long story short, I wasn't
allowed to go back to nursing, so I've been retired since 1993. I
miss it terribly. I miss the communication with people, but I find
with the church, and stuff like that, that I am still active and it sort
of compensates for it. I have my Theology of Ministry diploma
and I am a lay reader. I usually visit people in their homes and
pray with them and talk with them—especially the aging. It's very
interesting. It went together, the nursing and the ministry.

A personal success was when I received life membership in the
College of Registered Nurses Association. Nursing gave me a
lot. This need I had to help people was fulfilled. I always had a
really good relationship with people and I don't know if it all
came about because of my compassionate nature and the feeling
of caring. I believe strongly that a life is very, very important

and my husband, children and grandchildren make my life very worthwhile and fulfilling.

## ALFREDA DOUGLAS

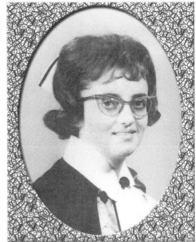

*Alfreda graduated from St. Elizabeth's Hospital in 1965. Shortly afterward, she joined the Royal Canadian Navy as a nursing sister. Alfreda enjoyed the travel and adventure of a military career. She has fond memories of her work with the Air Medical Evacuation Service. Alfreda retired in 1994 with health issues but has remained active in the Nursing Sisters Association.*

Even as a child, I wanted to be a nurse. You know, when you're going to school, they bring in career counsellors, say in Grade 11 or 12. I changed my mind a couple of times, but I came back to nursing.

I trained in a Catholic hospital and the sisters were firm with us but I think they needed to be. Still, I loved the training. I even enjoyed the first autopsy that I saw and that was within our first two months. Because we were in classes for two months and after that we were between classes and on the job training which is, I think, much better than what they do now. We went away to Halifax for our obstetrics course and the Infirmary and that was for three months. Our class was also the first to take psychiatric nursing. I soon discovered that psych nursing wasn't my forté. You have to be a special person, I think, to go into psych nursing and that wasn't me. Mine was pediatrics, obstetrics and the OR. We went to Point Edward for a month doing our TB nursing. As each year went by, we got a bit more responsibility and as seniors we were put in charge on weekends or on evening shifts.

When I graduated in '65, I spent a year working in pediatrics. I decided that summer that I wanted to join the navy, see the world. When I joined I went to Halifax initially. At that time, we were called nursing sisters. I worked part time at Camp Hill. In '67, I did my air med evacuation course at the base in Trenton, Ontario, that was about six weeks. Then I got posted to Comox, British Columbia. I got to travel on the Argus which was the precursor to the big aircraft that do patrols now. We got trained for nuclear accident responses. We went through exercises, had to dress in suits, they had to be washed down and then you had to check the Geiger count. That was quite an experience in itself.

We would be called out anytime, anywhere in the province of BC when a patient needed to be picked up from a hospital in the outer areas. We would take them down to Vancouver. One medevac I did at that time was the first set of Siamese twins I had ever seen. They were joined at the chest and the abdomen. Beautiful babies, but unfortunately they didn't survive. I went to Gagetown and spent two years there. While I was in Gagetown, I did one of our administrative courses—that was three months. You learned, as an officer, military procedure. My first position as a senior nurse was in Manitoba. I spent a year there. From there, I got transferred to Summerside, PEI. We travelled all over the Maritimes picking up patients. I always had a bag hanging in my office at the hospital. We would just grab it and go. We worked with Search and Rescue and they were just a fantastic group of people. I have a lot of respect for the job they are doing, because sometimes I used to get airsick. The one thing I never, ever wanted to do was go down from the helicopter to the ship—it was just a hoist—but I would sit and watch them, seeing the ship going up and down in the water and he's in the hoist going back and forth. Sometimes it was pretty rough but I did love doing air medevacs.

I lived in downtown Summerside, on the base, because I didn't drive at the time. Another American air force nurse who was posted there came and taught me how to drive so I got my first car and was able to move off the base. I left Summerside in '75 and went to Greenwood, Nova Scotia. Then I went to Ottawa from '78 to '82. That was my longest posting, a large hospital called the National Defence Medical Center. While I was there, I went to Germany on a three-month course to redo obstetrics. When I came back, I was transferred back to BC for three years.

The Argus was going to Hawaii on a trip so I asked if I could go. One of the other girls went too. I was allowed to go up in the cockpit. One of the pilots came back and I sat in his seat. I saw the Milky Way as we were flying. What a beautiful sight that was. We spent some time in Hawaii and went to San Francisco on the way back. We could stay in the American bases down there for 50¢ a night. On another trip, we went just outside of Disneyland in California. At that time the Vietnam war was still in progress. While I was there, one of the American aircrafts came in, one of those huge planes. It was just like walking into a hospital ward. It was so interesting to see that. I had some interesting times.

I became the first female president of the mess committee. That was one thing I enjoyed. The longer we stayed in, the more responsibility you got, which is the same as working in a civilian hospital. But the expectations were a little different in that you were told that you were an officer first. When I first joined the navy, our working uniform was blue, same as the army and we wore veils. In 1970, it became the Canadian Armed Forces. We all wore green. That was one thing I didn't like because we were all the same. Outside the hospital, we did not wear our working uniform. We changed into our street uniform.

I retired in 1994 due to my health. Now I belong to the Nursing Sisters Association. I'm on the visiting committee so we go once a month to visit the nursing sisters from the World War II. I keep in contact with a lot of my friends from right across the country and even in Germany. By joining the military, I had many different experiences, travelling and friendships.

## THELMA (TIMMONS) GRANT

*Thelma graduated from Sydney City Hospital in 1961 and nursed briefly in Sydney before marrying and starting a family. She returned to work full time in 1972 and spent most of her career at Harbour View Hospital in Sydney Mines. Thelma retired in 1994. She recalls the realities of shift work, living as a nurse in a rural community and the changes in health care she viewed first hand during three decades.*

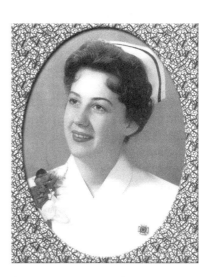

My mother always wanted to be a nurse, but way back then, you know, it wasn't possible for her to do that. When she was in her sixties she took a course and was a licenced practical nurse. She drove from Big Bras d'Or to MacGillivray Guest Home. She was there probably a year and a half or two years, but she loved it. These were probably some of the factors that influenced me. I just wanted to do it. I lived her vision.

I guess I was out of high school three years. I did some practice teaching. You were allowed to teach school with a permissive licence, in areas where they couldn't get a teacher. I did that for a year and I found out that it wasn't for me. Then I worked for a few years.

I was in training in September of 1958. We got paid once a month. I think the first year we got $10 a month. There was a spaghetti shop down on George Street, you got a dinner for 69¢ so we used to walk down and have that. There was a really close bond, you know, when you live with people for three years you get to know a lot about them. We still have our reunions and it's past forty years.

Right after graduation I stayed at the City for two months and I worked in the emergency department. I got married and didn't work anymore, probably a few private duties. Our first child was born late the next year. Then our second child was born so I didn't go to work for any length of time until 1968. My husband was injured and I had to go. I worked sporadically until 1972 and I went on staff then. So the first ten years, I wasn't really doing a lot. But in a rural community, you always got calls that somebody was sick, somebody had a fever, got cut, fell. It was a busy, busy time. You always went because it was your neighbours or your relatives.

I had real trouble with the shift work, 7-to-3 was fine, 3-to-11 was okay but night shift.... I couldn't sleep in the daytime. It was really difficult. I worked in all the departments. It was a small general hospital. I loved all the children, but especially ages one to six and I loved emergency. The old Harbour View in Sydney Mines wasn't what they would call ideal today, but it was a wonderful place to work. Everybody helped each other and of course when we went to the new hospital, then it was a totally different ball game.

I always remember in my second year, on night shift, I had a boy who had been hit by a train in Sydney and they didn't know who he was. As little as I knew back then, I knew he was going to die. To me that was so tragic. He was identified after he died. I think he was ten or eleven. That's a long time ago, but that was a clear memory. When I came to work on the Northside, you would see a bad diagnosis, you had to carry that around with you because you couldn't talk to anybody about it. And in the hospital where I worked, living in a rural community, we would get many of my neighbours, friends. When the prognosis wasn't good, it was burdensome. The fact that you couldn't talk about it, you were just supposed to leave that there when you left work, but you know it was still in your head. We were taught to be stoic. You didn't exhibit any emotion. That changed, too, through the years. Many, many times we would shed tears with people.

Nursing was really patient-centered in the early years, you know, and it changed. You had to spend so much time with writing and documenting. There was always the thought of your liability. We saw two court cases where patients had died. You know, it was a pretty scary experience. We saw a change, too, in the treatment of patients. They were encouraged to be mobile so much earlier and of course new medications. There were lots of changes, but none of it hit you "bang," like that. It was all phased in. You came along with it. I was always interested in furthering my education. They must have gotten tired of seeing my name on applications to attend workshops. If there was something you could learn to help somebody, then it was good to have it. Even at my age, I'm learning something new every day.

I received an award in 1985. I was Nurse of the Year for Cape Breton-Victoria. It's a long time ago, but it was quite a thrill. The last twelve years I worked in the veterans unit, extended care. You knew they were going to be with you for the duration. It was really important to keep a good relationship. I was there to help them to health or to help them toward the end. Your satisfaction is in comfort. So if you comfort someone following surgery and you saw them mobilize and you discharge them for home, that was one thing. But then if you had someone who was terminally ill, to comfort them or help them in their lonely times, that was fully as important as to help that other person get well.

I retired in 1994. It was time. You know, when you get to be in your fifties, it's hard work and at that point I was working at the DVA unit in Sydney Mines and it was very heavy work. It takes its toll on you, on your body. Just before I retired, the degree program was in the process of getting established here. It should be an advantage. It certainly gives a lot of exposure to stuff we didn't get. It will be interesting to see what's going to take place.

1966: The new Harbour View Hospital opened.

# VICTORIA COUNTY

## NEIL'S HARBOUR

### JESSIE (KAVANAUGH) CURTIS
As told by her daughter Bette Curtis
Connolly

*B*ette Curtis Connolly of Dartmouth
*shares her memories of her mother's
nursing career in Sydney and Ingonish.
Jessie was a community nurse who
played a vital role in her city and rural
neighbourhoods. She worked on the
scene of the Halifax Explosion and
through the Great Depression. Her
daughter's pride is evident as she recalls
her mother's nursing duties.*

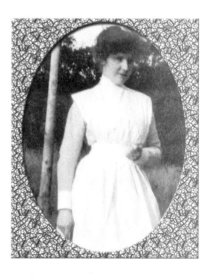

Jessie Kavanaugh was born in 1898 in Dominion. She completed
her high school education and, as she was too young to enroll in
nursing in Nova Scotia and rather than sit out a year, she went
to Boston to live with her aunt and train as a registered nurse at
the Boston City Hospital. She graduated in 1916, after which she
returned to Nova Scotia and settled in Sydney. There, she joined
the Victorian Order of Nurses. She married Doane Curtis in 1918.

She pursued a career in nursing because it was her goal in life. She especially loved working with children and the elderly. In those early years, there were not many nurses around. Ashby was a very close-knit community and it was also Depression time and not much money available. If there was a nurse in the community, she would be called on to do a variety of nursing duties for her neighbours. During our growing-up years, she delivered many of the neighbourhood babies. As my father worked twelve-hour shifts at the Sydney steel plant, it was not unusual for an expectant father to babysit us and walk the floor while she would go to his house and deliver their baby. I recall on one occasion, twins were born, but only one was expected. She came home after the delivery, cut diapers out of two flannel sheets and hemmed them so they would have enough diapers for two. On another occasion, my sister had a group of young friends at the house. One of them went home and told his mother where he had been. She told him that Mrs. Curtis had delivered him. He was quite excited about this and came to visit her the next day.

One of the most memorable experiences she had was during the Halifax Explosion, which happened on December 6, 1917. There was an urgent call for nurses. A gentleman volunteered to drive any nurses who would go to Halifax. My mother and one other nurse volunteered and it took them two days to get from Sydney to Halifax. The roads were bad, there was no Canso Causeway. Cars were taken across by ferry. The trains were also shunted on the ferry.

My father was from Ingonish, where my grandmother operated a hotel. The family spent two months there every summer. When word got around she was there, people would come to the door looking for advice. I remember a man came to the door with a little boy crying in pain. The father was sure he was having an appendix attack. She checked it out, gave him an enema and he was fine. They were forever grateful. While we were there, she also volunteered to visit elderly people and do things to make them feel better like cutting fingernails, toenails, etc. Dr. C. H. MacMillan, who had a practice in Baddeck, also made calls in Ingonish. He stayed in the hotel and often called on my mother to assist him. The dining room table was his examination table.

She was very proud of her uniform: the cap which identified
the hospital she graduated from, the full-length white uniform
starched to perfection and her navy cape with red satin lining, as
well as the VON blue uniform with the navy blue coat and hat.
She was devastated on her first stay in hospital after the nurses
had won the right not to wear uniforms. When a nurse came into
her room in a sweat suit, she had to be convinced she was really
a nurse. During a stay myself at the Victoria General Hospital a
few years ago, a nurse came into my room with a nurse's cap and
beautiful uniform. I immediately thought of my mother and told
her: "If my mother could see this, she would be very pleased."

## HANNAH (MacDONALD) MATHESON
As told by a source who wishes to
remain anonymous

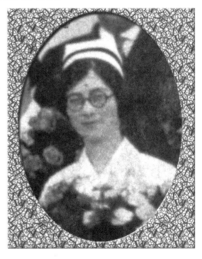

*Hannah was born and raised on
the North Shore of Victoria
County. In 1922, she moved to Boston,
graduating from the school of nursing
at the Massachusetts State Infirmary in
1925. Hannah worked in Boston until
1931, when she married and returned to
Cape Breton. For many years, she ran
a tourist home, raised her family and
served as a community nurse. When her
family moved to Sydney Mines in 1945,
Hannah continued to nurse in local
hospitals and opened her home to newly-released hospital patients from the
North Shore. She moved to Tatamagouche in 1968 and died in Halifax in
1988.*

Sarah Johannah, Hannah, was born on the North Shore at Plaster
in 1902. She completed her early education at North Shore
and acquired her senior matriculation at Baddeck. In 1922, she
enrolled in the school of nursing at the Mass State Infirmary
in Tewksbury, Massachusetts. Upon graduation, she worked in
several Boston hospitals and did special duty with many patients
in their homes. It was during this time Hannah brought her
widowed mother and young family to Boston, where she helped

support them. In the early 1930s, the entire family moved to Detroit, Michigan.

In 1931, Hannah married and returned to Cape Breton where she and her husband took up residence on the family farm. In the late 1930s, they turned the family home into a tourist home and Hannah filled a busy role of hostess, mother, homemaker and community nurse. She was on constant community call for the sick and country maternity cases in the area. Sometimes, she would be gone from her home for several days if it was a slow delivery. At her funeral, one lady told Hannah's son that Hannah delivered eight of her children.

When the Matheson family moved to Sydney Mines in 1945, Hannah continued to do special duty, fulfilling her role at both Harbour View Hospital and St. Elizabeth's Hospital in North Sydney. In Sydney Mines, the Matheson home became a haven for patients from the country who would convalesce there after release from the hospital and before returning to their own homes. Sometimes they would be with Hannah and her husband for two weeks or more.

In 1968, Hannah and her husband moved to Tatamagouche to be near their family. Hannah was a nurse until the day she died. She would have made a wonderful doctor. She seemed to have a firm understanding of medicine and such a compassionate way of dealing with the sick in body and heart. She died in 1988 and is buried in Breton Cove, Cape Breton.

Hannah's obituary in her community newspaper describes her dedication to her profession:

> ...Hannah was a registered nurse and lived in our community at a time when her skill and knowledge was much needed. Time and again she was called upon to serve when there was sickness, terminal illness, accidents and births. She would always respond with compassion and competent care, dressed in the uniform of a profession she served with honor. Wherever there was sickness or suffering, just knowing Hannah was coming made things seem better....

## EMILY (MACLEAN) MACLEOD
As told by her son Bill MacLeod

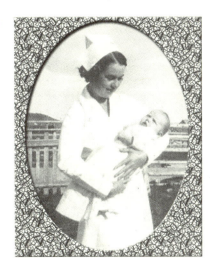

*Emily graduated from the Salvation Army Grace Maternity Hospital in Halifax in 1935 with training in obstetrics and child care. She was assigned to the Salvation Army Hospital in Sydney as a private nurse. Emily resigned in 1940 to start her family. She moved to Ingonish and nursed in that community for many years. Her son Bill remembers her impact on families and community as well as her pride in her profession.*

Mother had several reasons for becoming a nurse. She was the eldest of three siblings. Her father was a clergyman and her parents were very busy. She was required to look after the younger children. Her mother had some health problems and that made Emily's help even more essential. After high school graduation, she worked for a time as a companion to a doctor's wife. It was after seeking counsel from that doctor that she decided to become a maternity/newborn nurse.

Emily had fond memories of her education program. It was very strict, but supportive. All students lived at the hospital residence. Time allowed outside of the hospital was limited because they worked and studied long hours. They had to respect a strict curfew. Uniforms, including shoes, were to be worn in the hospital only. Street clothes were never worn inside. She had a deep respect for the Salvation Army and what it was accomplishing. Doctors and matrons were superiors and were treated very respectfully. If students were seated when a doctor or matron entered the room, the students were to stand as a sign of respect.

One of Emily's fond memories during her education was her private duty nursing. She would stay by the bed of her patient and minister to her needs. She formed strong friendships during her time at the Grace. She corresponded with a fellow student for over fifty years. Emily graduated first in her class. Top standing was very important to her.

After graduation, Emily worked at the Salvation Army Hospital in Sydney. Once again she made strong bonds with staff and patients. One of the patients who later required close nursing attention became a lifelong friend and, later, so did her family. Today, although Emily and the patient are both deceased, their children maintain those strong ties.

She delighted in the births of the babies. It did distress her when a baby was lost. Even fifty years later, she would cry when relating the story of a beautiful baby who was stillborn. Forty years after leaving her position at the hospital in Sydney, she was stopped by a lady in a Sydney store. The woman said she would never forget her because of the wonderful care she received as her patient in the hospital in the 1930s. For us, her children, Mother's dedication was noted to us at her memorial service.

She resigned from her nursing position at the hospital in Sydney in late 1940. At that time she was interested in starting her own family. Upon moving to Ingonish, she was still active in the community for many years, assisting at births and providing other nursing care. There was not always a doctor available. Sometimes she assisted the doctor at the birth, other times she handled the delivery alone. She also helped out in the community when medical assistance was required, changing bandages, administering insulin shots, etc.

One particularly memorable incident involved an infant who could not keep down his formula, threw up violently and steadily lost weight. It was winter and there was lots of ice and snow and no doctor was near. Upon conferring with a doctor in Sydney, it was determined this was a life and death situation and the infant should be evacuated by plane to North Sydney. The plane landed on the ice covering Warren Lake and Emily and the baby were settled into the front seat of the two-seat plane while the pilot occupied the seat directly behind them. They landed at Kelly's Beach where the doctor was waiting and they were transported to the hospital. The baby was treated successfully and he and nurse Emily returned to Ingonish and the child's grateful parents in the spring. That baby is now a retired grandfather of seven. Nurse MacLean was made an associate member of the Cape Breton Flying Club for one day. The sick infant was the youngest passenger they ever transported.

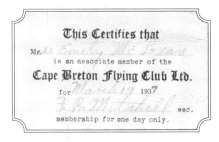

This Certifies that

Mr. *Emily Mc Lean*

is an associate member of the

**Cape Breton Flying Club Ltd.**

for *March 19* 1937

*F. B. Mitchell* sec.

membership for one day only.

Babies set their own timetable. It was not unusual for her to be called out any hour of the day or night and sometimes in very bad weather. More than once she travelled by horse and sleigh through heavy snow. Emily's uniforms were very important to her. Her white hat and dresses were always kept clean, starched and ironed. Even when delivering babies in Ingonish, she wore her uniform.

In later years, she felt that nurses carried a much heavier load than they did when she was practising. In one way, she felt that it was unfortunate because the nurses are so busy, they no longer have the time to provide the extra little personal touches that so many patients appreciate.

---

1943: The North Victoria Cottage Hospital opened at Neil's Harbour.

1945: A group of Victoria County residents began planning to provide hospital facilities to cater to the medical needs of about 5,000 residents. Funds were raised through public subscription and the Victoria County Memorial Hospital was constructed in Baddeck at a cost of $104,000. It opened in 1949, debt free. The Canadian Red Cross ran the hospital for the first five years.

1950: Wilhelmina (Creelman) MacDonald was appointed administrator of Victoria County Memorial Hospital. She retired in 1978.

1953: The new Buchanan Memorial Hospital opened in Neil's Harbour.

1966: The community of Neil's Harbour built a home and office in an effort to attract a doctor.

1974: A new pediatric wing was constructed at Buchanan Memorial at a cost of $105,985.

---

## Sharon (Donovan) Williams

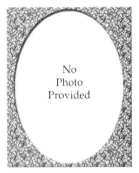

No
Photo
Provided

*Sharon graduated from St. Elizabeth's Hospital in 1966. She worked briefly at large hospitals, but spent most of her career at the small community hospital in Neil's Harbour. Sharon ended her career in a geriatric setting and retired in 2001. She remembers the variety of a rural nursing career and also the heavy responsibilities.*

I thought nursing would be great. I sat with my grandfather while he was dying and I was familiar with sick people. I wasn't frightened of it. I was incredibly young when I entered training; seventeen in September—in October of that year I was on the floor. On the floor meant passing out trays and you got involved with the patient. Giving out trays then meant you set it up and you sat with them, not like today where the tray is given out by kitchen staff. We worked very hard and we were used for service but the responsibility we were given is amazing. My third year meant I was alone on the floor on back shift and I was in charge of it. The start of my second year, I was in the back of an ambulance from North Sydney to Sydney with a young man in a motorcycle accident who was paralyzed from the neck down. I did all that and didn't bat an eyelash. We were a very close class, about thirty of us.

When I graduated, I was ready to nurse, I was ready to take on anything. I still felt I had a lot to learn and every day I learned something new. I think that is why a lot of graduates now only work for so many years and leave it because they are very disillusioned. If they spent six months in a hospital, wide open during training, they would know if they liked it or not.

I worked at the VG and I worked in Newfoundland, in the OR in these places. I hated working in the operating room at the Victoria General because there was no hands-on. I scrubbed for open heart surgery one time, very fascinating but I always like hands-on nursing. My two favourite types of nursing, especially in Neil's Harbour, were maternity and cardiac care. They were so intense and then, of course, joyful. Every delivery was different. You were very close to the mother. It made me feel I was part of the community. The cardiac care, they were next to death, of course, and you did everything you could to get them back on their feet again. They were definitely my favourites.

I went to Neil's Harbour in 1967, no doubt it was my favourite. You become very involved with the people, with the patient and their families. I spent many an hour on the ambulance because then we transferred many of the patients to Sydney or Halifax. If I worked a shift and there was someone there to go, I went. The highlight of my career was looking after a five year-old boy who died at home with a brain tumour. I slept beside him and I looked after him for a few months before he died. I looked after many people in their own homes. We did it all.

You experience heartache in your career every time there is a death, especially people you are very close with in the community. Having a stillborn was devastating. I have been with many that didn't survive: car accidents, cardiac patients. You had to be there for all the family, we did not have a crisis team to call in.

It is very difficult, but it is amazing how you learn and how you grow. You are able to do that. I found if you showed your feelings, if you cried and they cried, they felt they had someone they could rely on at that moment. The nurses were very good. They did not go home and talk about patients. That was hammered into us and was extremely important. You had to be very careful; when I started in Neil's Harbour, we were on a party line.

It is teamwork: teamwork with the doctor, the other nurses, the dietician, the cleaning staff, everyone, and it is especially important in a nursing home. When you know these people, it is difficult, no matter how tired you are. You've got to be able to smile once in a while. If you don't have time, it is difficult to be happy and smile. I ended my career working in long term care and geriatrics and I can honestly say, no matter how difficult long term care was, that was one of my most rewarding. I retired in 2001. I wasn't feeling well. I have missed it. My whole life is nursing.

I see a major evolution in nursing. The uniform wasn't for the nurse, it was for the patient. I still believe to this day, if the patient could see the uniform with the black band it was very comforting because they knew they had the RN, not the cleaning lady. Now you don't know who you got. There are times that I get a wee bit scared of getting old and to think of what nursing will be. We are going to have an extreme shortage of nurses.

## REGINA (DONOVAN) WILLIAMS

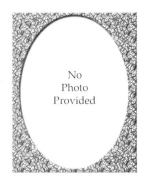

*Regina graduated from St. Rita Hospital in 1979 and began her career in cardiac care at the Victoria General in Halifax. She moved home to Neil's Harbour a year later and spent twenty-three years in the small community hospital. Regina and her husband also ran a tourist business and she retired in 2001 to devote her time to family and the business. Regina has fond memories of nursing in a small community.*

Nursing is something I wanted all my life. I enjoyed people and I just always wanted to make someone feel better. I found the training wonderful. We weren't even there that long when we started going out on the floors so we got a lot of actual hands-on work. When it was such a short course you had to get out and start right away. But the training was excellent. It was very concentrated. Looking back, it seemed that we were very young to come out with the responsibilities that we did. I turned twenty and, five days later, I graduated. It just seemed like there wasn't much life experience there. I was a country girl who was very sheltered all her life. It almost seems like we should have been older, going out to accept that responsibility. At the time you are young and cocky and you don't think anything of it; now I look back and think: "Oh my God."

When I first finished training, I went to the Victoria General Hospital and they put me through cardiac training. I stayed there for a year before I transferred back home. I loved cardiac care. Working as a nurse in a small hospital, I found you had a lot more responsibility than in the bigger hospitals, because 90 per cent of the time we had no doctor. There was always a doctor on call, but there was never a doctor that stays in the hospital 24/7. We did a lot of things I didn't do when I was at the VG. Our doctors started doing things with us and we'd do it three times. Then they would say whether we were capable of doing it on our own. They trained us for things like starting IVs and EKGs. If you had someone in the middle of the night taking chest pains, we don't have round the clock lab techs so simple blood work—like if someone took a heart attack and you wanted to do cardiac enzymes in the first hour—we would draw the blood and just refrigerate it until the lab came in. I just found we learned more and did more, after we had the teaching. It was wonderful and made us feel more confident. We knew the doctor wasn't always going to be available. Time can be of the essence.

I really enjoyed my time in delivery. We used to do all our deliveries here in Neil's Harbour, but we've since given it up. We had between thirty and forty births a year. It is a joyful thing to be going through labour and delivery when all goes well. You learn from everybody in the community. You may not know some of the patients, but there was definitely some of the family you would know. It was nice, but at times it could be difficult too. If someone was dying, it was hard to stay objective, but the level of caring in our little hospital was wonderful.

Since it is a small community, if someone gets sick, through the grapevine everyone knows it within twenty minutes, so you never really had to worry that you were going to disclose something because everybody knew everything anyway. It would come on the scanner if an ambulance was called to someone's house and what was going on.

I also did work for a couple of years part-time in the nursing home here in Neil's Harbour, which I really enjoyed. I loved the old folks and it was a lot of bedside nursing. My least favourite to work in would be pediatrics. I just cannot deal with a sick kid. I am just too emotional with a child. Our hospital continually offered courses. They encouraged you to go and take them to keep up with your knowledge. They kept us well updated. Uniforms were more important in the bigger hospital, I found. Down here, in the smaller one, it seemed like everybody knew all the nurses anyway so you didn't need a white uniform to stand out, for them to know this is the nurse. I think the changes in uniforms make people more relaxed, especially around children, it's not so scary. I don't think it hurt at all coming from the community and going back and working in the community hospital. I think it made people feel even more comfortable with you.

Looking back on my nursing years, I enjoyed it. The last few years, I didn't care for it as much. It seems like we are getting away from the actual hands-on care that we used to do. It's becoming more of a professional job instead of a nurturing job. I guess, to me, the whole aspect of it has changed. Computers and technology is wonderful. It can save lives in an instant when you can have access to doctors you are four hours away from, and that's wonderful, but it takes away from the actual patient-nurse relationship and I enjoyed my time spent at the bedside. The last few years I worked, I didn't find I had the time to be there.

I retired three years ago. My husband and I owned our own business in Ingonish. It's a tourist operation, so from May to November, I'm extremely busy. I had four children in under five years. I just thought that going out and working all night, coming home and being tired and strung out, just wasn't worth it. It was taking away from my family life. I enjoyed being home with my kids. After I had the last one, I went back just part-time.

I think the sky is the limit with the nursing today. It is so much more advanced than the training when I was in it. I came out not owing a cent. Today, if you have to borrow, you are looking at at least $40,000. How do you start out owing that kind of money?

# INVERNESS COUNTY

1923: Inverness Memorial Hospital was founded as a memorial to citizens who lost their lives in World War I. It opened with 12 beds. Staff included Dr. P. S. Cochrane, Miss Jessie Woodbury, RN, two graduate nurses, a maid and a caretaker.

1929: An addition to the hospital was announced.

## RITA (JONES) SMITH
As told to Betty MacLean

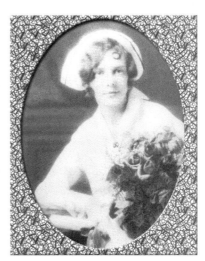

*Rita graduated from Sydney City Hospital School of Nursing in 1930 and worked there for a few years before moving to Inverness. In Inverness, Rita married and continued nursing at the hospital until her first child was born. She continued private duty nursing and helped her husband run a community general store. Rita moved to Dartmouth after her husband's death in 1980. In 2003, she shared her nursing memories with her "niece" Betty MacLean. Rita died in May of 2004.*

Rita was born in Wales in 1905 and came to Canada in 1908. Her parents raised five children in Whitney Pier. In 1927, Rita entered nurse's training at Sydney City Hospital. The head nurse was always on her case for talking and laughing. They were not even permitted to smile in class.

Rita graduated in 1930 and worked at Sydney City Hospital for a period, however, in 1932 a request came from the Inverness Hospital which had lost the services of a nurse and she went on loan from Sydney to Inverness Memorial. In 1933, she married and remained in Inverness where her husband operated a general store. Rita continued nursing until 1935, when their daughter was born. In those days, when a woman became pregnant, she was not permitted to remain in the work force. Rita did, however, continue private duty nursing. While in Inverness, there was a woman who was quite ill before the birth of her baby and had to be in hospital. Rita was doing private duty nursing for the family. After the birth of her baby the woman was very worried and every time she heard a baby crying in the nursery she would beg Rita to ensure her baby was not in distress. Rita was frequently sent off to see if the baby was crying. After many false alarms, in desperation, Rita would pick up the quietest baby, put the blanket up just to expose the baby's face a bit and show it to the mother to prove it was not crying. This satisfied the woman. It was not until many years later that Rita told her the difference.

In 1942, a son was born. Rita remained at home to care for the children and also assisted her husband in the family business. She was called on occasionally to do private nursing within the community.

When her husband passed away, Rita and her son moved to Dartmouth to be near her daughter. Rita remained active in the community through involvement with choir. She enjoyed travelling and visited several countries, including Wales, as well as visiting family and friends in Canada and the United States. Rita was an avid bridge player and continued until her eyesight failed to the extent that she could no longer read the cards.

Sometime in 2003, Rita and I were talking about the good old days. I explained that the Retired Nurses Association was looking for stories from former nursing trainees and was planning a book. Rita was more than willing to have her story submitted.

Rita will ever be in my memory. We shared many happy adventures ... one of her favourites was the "wash and wax" machine we went through, in the car of course. Rita was fascinated by this bit of modern technology. It was always a joy to be in her company.

> 1931: Cheticamp founded its first hospital with the help of Les filles des Jesus, a religious order based in Quebec.

## ROBERTA (MACMILLAN) CAMERON

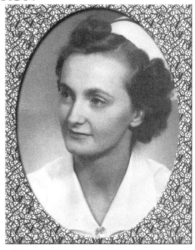

*Roberta graduated from the Halifax Infirmary in 1941 and remained on staff there for five years, on the merchant marine ward. After the war, she returned to her native Inverness, married and raised nine children. Roberta managed to continue nursing while she raised her family, sometimes doing private duty and later as a staff nurse at the local hospital. She retired in 1979. At age 85, Roberta has vivid memories of her training and wartime experiences and of advances in health care.*

Coming out of school there seemed to be two options for a young girl in Inverness then: you are going into training or going into teaching. I have an older sister who was a teacher and in those days the younger sister would come in and substitute. I was sixteen when I would go there, and all I could do was tell stories to keep them in their seats. I said I would not be able to keep discipline in the classroom so I will go into training. My father was a doctor, but he had died when I was four so I was always interested in things like that.

Off I went to Halifax and it was the first time I was ever on a train. I must say, I enjoyed the training and loved the hospital and those who taught me; it was the Sisters of Charity. They were very thorough teachers and very conscientious, very kind. I took my training in the nursery, case room, the OR. The last part of my training was on the merchant marine ward—all the seamen who came in ill or wounded! And there were plenty of them. I got a terrific experience then and I asked to work on that ward when I went on staff after I graduated. When I wrote my RNs, I led the province.

I stayed there for five years. I became acquainted with many people from all over the world; from China, India, France, even Russians came in at that time. It was quite a broadening experience. Medically, it was terrific: we had tropical fevers—they came in with malaria and sometimes we were overcrowded and had beds in the corridor—you get the smell of tobacco and old sea bags; there might be five, six or seven survivors of the torpedoing; we had survivors of a ship with a bunch of young boys—they had a machine gun and were shooting at the U-boats. They were just full of shrapnel.

Many times we spent months just healing broken bones and wounds. At that time all the new drugs came out, penicillin and others. I will never forget soludagamin, an intramuscular injection. It was an antibiotic. These four Russian men came in; they had meningitis which at that time was fatal. They were delirious. Their shoulders were chafed with the skin off them from tossing to and fro in their beds. The doctor came and I will always remember the red solution. He gave it to them intramuscularly and within 48 hours their temperatures were normal. We were just absolutely amazed at the power of those drugs.

After the war, we came home and got married. I went on staff at the Inverness Memorial Hospital and I worked there off and on. At that time, if you weren't on staff, you were on private duty and you were always in demand because if anybody had an operation and wanted to have a special nurse sit by them and pamper them, that was my role. It was good for me because I had to do it in between children. I had nine children. When I became pregnant, I would stay home for awhile and I had help at home so I would go back. It didn't hurt them because they all became good parents themselves. I carried on until I was sixty. That would be about 1979.

It was always a joy to see someone recover from a horrible illness or injury. In the day's work, the hardest was keeping the charts up. I would keep running around until the last minute trying to remember what you did and your medications and everything. I have seen myself starting to walk into town because I am two miles out of town. If it was morning, I could call in and say I can't make it, but if you were working 3-to-11 on the floor in the little hospital, there would be one RN and one aid on the floor. You could not not turn up. Sometimes I would have to walk and hail the first car coming. I don't care if you are Jack The Ripper, I have to get to the hospital. They would always get me there safe.

The care we gave to the patient was very good. Now, the medical people think it is better to let the patient do it themselves as soon as they open their eyes. We used to bathe them, rub their back, their feet, clean their nails, braid their hair. It took quite a while to do each patient in the morning.

## ALICE (MACLEAN) FREEMAN

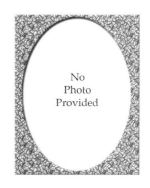

No Photo Provided

*Alice graduated from Glace Bay General in 1958. She began a 30-year career at Inverness Hospital where she worked in all departments and as a head nurse. When Alice retired in 1988, she opened a small business in her community. She remembers the great variety of nursing in a small community hospital and the health care changes she saw through the decades.*

I spent time in the hospital as a child and I thought the nurses looked spiffy in their white uniforms and caps. I received my nursing education at Glace Bay General Hospital. I was eighteen years old when I entered in 1955. For four months leading up to my enrollment, I worked in the hospital as a nurse's aid.

I enjoyed my training, although at this time the hospital ran things like the military and we were told not to get too close with the patients. We were well trained and prepared. On my first shift I delivered a baby.

As part of general duty in Inverness you worked in all departments, plus I worked as Medicine Control until the pharmacy opened. Then I was head nurse for the ten years prior to retirement. When someone came up to me years later and told me what I did for them, I knew I was appreciated. As head nurse, I thought it was important to push my staff to further their education and knowledge through workshops, reading and meeting nurses from other hospitals.

It was a joy to see a patient who was sick go home. It was difficult when a family member was upset that he or she wasn't notified of a family member's death. Legally the hospital is to only call the person listed by the patient as next of kin. We once had an incident where a daughter was not informed of her mother's death by the hospital and was quite irate with us. She didn't understand that her mother did not have her listed as next of kin and the other person we had notified had not called her.

My most memorable accomplishment was as head nurse of Inverness Hospital, I worked with the head nurse of St. Mary's Hospital to help amalgamate the staff when we moved into the new Inverness Consolidated Hospital.

Uniforms were very important to me. Today, you can't tell the cleaning staff from the nurses. There must be some way they can be identified, perhaps having the nurses wear their black band on their uniforms.

I retired in 1987, as I was professionally burnt out. In 1988, I opened my own business.

I see very little nursing care or bedside nursing by the RN's as there is too much paperwork. I would like to see nurses going back to bedside nursing and looking after patients.

## MARY LEE (WATERS) MORRISON AND TINA (MATTHEWS) WATERS
Joint Interview

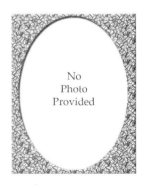

No
Photo
Provided

*Tina graduated from Sydney City Hospital in 1960 and began her career at the Inverness Hospital. She retired in 1999 but returned to work a few years later as a casual. Mary Lee graduated from the Victoria General Hospital in 1962 and also nursed in Inverness, retiring in 1989. In a joint interview, they remember the joys and*

*heartaches of working in a small community hospital, harrowing winter
driving and the changes they've seen in their profession.*

Mary Lee:

I went to Dal for a couple of years and then the VG. I had never
really been away from home that much. It's a good thing I really
liked training. I always wanted to be a nurse. From training I went
right to Inverness and started in general duty. I was just a staff
nurse. The head nurses, I had so much respect for them. I thought:
"These nurses are getting old." I was only there about ten years
and I was with them. I was one of the older nurses because the
new ones started to come. We were just like one family. I had a
bit of trouble when I had my kids. It wasn't that easy to do both. I
always enjoyed obstetrics and I didn't like the OR. The paperwork
became a real nuisance as far as I was concerned. A lot of it has
become an administrative thing rather than bedside nursing.
But when people go into nursing now, they know what they are
getting into, I'm sure.

Tina:

I think I was a patient at the Sydney City Hospital in Grade 2. I
used to look at those nurses in their white, starched uniforms and
from there I wanted to be a nurse. I loved my training right from
the start. I was scared of a couple of head nurses. I went to work in
the OR at Sydney City after graduation. I went to Inverness after
that, just general duty. From there I was a supervisor for years.
I enjoyed working at the little hospital because I found we got
so much experience there. I think the hardest thing was getting
there on a stormy night, travelling in the winter by yourself. In
those days you had to have chains on your car and I remember
them breaking on the way and having to get under when I was
pregnant. There was no salt on the roads. I always minded the
deaths. I never, ever conquered that. I retired in 1999 and was
home for three years. I just went back last May, just casual. I
thought I'd go another little while yet. The roles are certainly
changing and they have been for awhile. Even today, for a nurse to
be sitting at a desk and a doctor to come, I feel like I should stand.
But they don't expect that anymore, either.

## Betty Jane Cameron

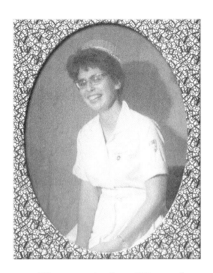

*Betty Jane graduated from McGill University in Montreal in 1961 and went on to complete a Master's Degree in Health Administration and Epidemiology. She taught and nursed, primarily in midwifery and mental health in the Caribbean, the U.S. and remote areas of Canada before settling in Inverness to raise her family. She retired in 1994 and now works as a music teacher. Her nursing adventures illustrate the diversity of the profession.*

I had an elderly cousin who was a nurse. She was in her 80s and always encouraged me to be a nurse. I went for the university course because I had been sick and my doctor said I would not be able to stand the three-year training. Little did he know I went in for five years. It was a wonderful course, the first of its kind. We worked eleven months a year for five years and we did university courses. As the years went on, we did maybe three days a week of practical work and two days of classes. We did supervisory and public health. We had a much wider experience than others did at the time. You met some wonderful people. Margaret Meade, an anthropologist, came and did a series of lectures. We all met her and spent time with her. Nobody thought we were nurses because we had to wear ugly royal blue uniforms and brown Oxfords. Everybody else would be wearing white. Patients would ask us to go get a nurse when they needed help. A couple of years later, I did my Master's in health administration, epidemiology and public health. I also earned my midwifery diploma.

I went back to McGill and taught, but the two years in between I worked at the Royal Victoria Hospital, Montreal, in maternity and then gynecological services. I did clinical instruction to the students there. There were seven nurseries. If you wanted a job, you just asked, there were jobs everywhere. I had a chance to go to Trinidad to nurse just because my friend in psychiatry didn't want the job. She asked me if I wanted it, no interviews. Nobody cared about my qualifications. People today don't get those kind of opportunities.

In Trinidad, we were dressed like ancient British nurses with the great big white, stiff veils and those dreadful white uniforms with the big elastic belts. I had a motorcycle and was called the "flying nun." There was a leprosarium. It was on a separate island that was a two hour ride from the mainland. The boat only went there once a week. It took doctors and supplies and they held a clinic there. People who were there, were there for life. It was awful because there were children born there. Some of them developed leprosy. That was extremely hard to see. I worked as director of the psychiatric hospital's school of nursing and helped set up modern care practices and educational standards for affiliations between psychiatric and general hospitals. I also worked with the World Health Organization to develop a nursing curriculum for the Southern Caribbean countries.

I worked in all kinds of places: Trinidad, Kentucky, northern Canada, Montreal, Halifax. I worked with wonderful people everywhere. People were much the same. When I was up north in a nursing station in Labrador, I talked to my mother and told her how the telephone had to operate, the radio phone. We could not carry on a dual conversation, it had to be two separate ones. Months later, I was delivering a mother in northern Newfoundland and she asked me how my mother was. Everyone up and down the coast heard my conversations.

I was working for the International Grenfell Association and Dalhousie University to set up a midwifery program. We were also responsible for the weather forecast three times a day. Basically, we would look up at the Mounties' clothesline and the flag to see what direction the wind was blowing. It was critical to get the right directions because most of our transportation was through airplanes. Many of the nursing stations were in remote harbours or just off the Atlantic. You had to know how the winds were blowing because planes made split second decisions about which way they were going to land safely. In the winter, if we were travelling on the only road in northern Newfoundland, we would take carloads of people who were waiting to go home to their little communities. People would come up to meet us if it was storming. Sometimes, they would come out with snow plows to get us safely back and Ski-Doos to bring us in. It was good to be around people like that.

Back in the hills of Kentucky, communications were different again, that was hillbilly country and they were still fighting over moonshine and property rights and old family feuds. We would get around on horseback with our saddlebags and our medical supplies on one side and deliver supplies on the other. I can remember once a man stopped me and asked me where I was going. I told him. He said: "Okay go straight ahead and don't take any side paths. He shot two shots up in the air saying okay, let me through. We were well protected by everybody if we were nurses.

Delivering a baby was always a miracle and watching someone die peacefully was a miracle. I always like the hands-on, clinical work. Even when I worked as director of care, when codes went off, and I was around, I would do my part in the resuscitation and I think the staff respected that I worked with them.

I was on my way from Dalhousie to work in northern Newfoundland and I met my husband in Mabou when I came through this corner of Inverness. So that is how I got here. I did go up to northern Newfoundland for a couple of years, but when I came back we were married. I stayed home to raise our children and then I got a job at Inverness Hospital. I did a lot of community nursing here. I retired in 1994 because they were downsizing the hospital. They did away with my position as director of patient care. I am a music teacher now. I also volunteer with community health care, pastoral care, the fire department and the Northwood Lifeline Program.

I think nursing has a good future, but I think we have to get back to the basics of listening to people because we don't often have the time, or take the time. The roles and responsibilities of nursing have changed dramatically. I think the future of nursing is safe and bright.

# Janice Ferguson

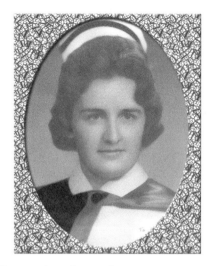

*Janice graduated from St. Joseph's in 1964. She spent most of her career in obstetrics at the Inverness Community Hospital, retiring in 1997. She is still active as a volunteer in her community. Janice recalls the joy of witnessing new life, the heartache of death and the special pleasures of nursing in a small community. She reflects on the changes in her profession and the future of nursing care.*

Nursing was just something I wanted to do and liked. My aunt tells me that from the time I was little, I was always doing something with someone. I graduated from high school in 1961 and went into training at the age of eighteen. We had an elective and that was obstetrics for me. The rest was general duty. I was an only girl and I distinctly remember my first night. I had to undress in front of my roommate so I hid and went into the closet to do it. My roommate at the time had a sister, so she wasn't shy.

In my training class there were two senior and two junior male nurses. Many of the times they were treated as orderlies or porters and were expected to lift, drag and pull. They are stronger, but they are nurses. Some patients would say they didn't want them looking after them, but I would remind them "your doctor is male." The old prejudice is still there. Every male nurse I worked with was caring and compassionate and a very good nurse. A lot of people treated them as if they were gay because they were in a woman's profession.

When I came home after my training was finished, I had applied to three or four hospitals for work and got accepted by all. This left me with a decision to make. I remember it was October 7 that I started working at St. Mary's Hospital in Inverness. From that day until the day I retired, I loved every day of it, there was always something new and challenging.

I absolutely loved mothers and babies and I didn't mind sick children. I think I truly liked obstetrics as not that much went wrong. I really loved old people. There were some old men at the hospital that were cranky and for some reason we got along really well. At the beginning of my career I worked on first floor, but the kitchen was on second so I would need to go up and make my patients their food and then bring it down. After they ate, the dishes needed to be washed, you had to make your own dressings and formulas for the babies in obstetrics and pediatrics We were running up and down the floors and borrowing off other departments for supplies and sharpening syringes before we got disposables.

At one time a doctor came up for a consultation, saying he was mindboggled by the knowledge of the nurses at Inverness Hospital. He said you could ask them anything. If they didn't know, you could be sure they would find out. Recently, when I was having surgery at the Victoria General in Halifax, one of the nurses commented that her son had received treatment in Inverness. She worked in a specialty for many years and she was boggled in all that we had to know as nurses and all that we had to do. During my career, if there was a major accident, the nurses would automatically come in. I don't know about now, but they used to. That's what small community hospitals are about.

I know that I had a pink uniform and a green one. We wore caps for a long time but I think a cap doesn't make a nurse and they were more bothersome as they were always being knocked off leaning over patients or reaching for something. I do find in the larger hospitals you cannot distinguish the kitchen staff, housekeeping or nurses. That must be hard for a patient.

Heartaches would be mothers or their babies dying and people I really cared about dying or becoming ill. In a small hospital and town, you not only know someone as a patient, you know their family or someone connected to the patient. One time, I had a patient die that I was very close to and the patient in the next bed to her had said to me: "I don't know how you nurses can be so cold." I said to her: "then why am I crying?" Another time, a friend stopped me in the hall and asked how nurses do this, do we cry? All the time—you may not see us, but we do.

No matter what was going on, I could honestly say I enjoyed all my days of nursing as every day was interesting and challenging and I was always learning. Sometimes you would go home mad and tired as hell, but it was still interesting. I have received a lot of letters since I retired. At my retirement party, my present head nurse said that what stood out as far as she could see was my rapport with the Native people. They all call me the baby nurse and still come here looking for me. I remember asking one of them why they single me out and she said: "Because you treat us like we are not different." I replied that they were not. I met one of the elders early in my career and I was very impressed with him. He spoke English, French, Gaelic and Mi'kmaq, was a World War II veteran and had seven sons and one daughter. He told me so much about their history and culture and was never angry.

The emphasis now seems to be on documenting and charting but what happens to the patient? Who looks after things? I think they have to go back to a diploma in nursing. I know from experience that it takes a year to teach a nurse to be a nurse. They need practise in order to learn. They come out of their four-year degree and then they are put in a small hospital like Inverness and they are absolutely terrified. I don't remember being terrified. I knew enough to survive but now there is something missing: the basics and practice.

## JUDITH (FERGUSON) GILLIS

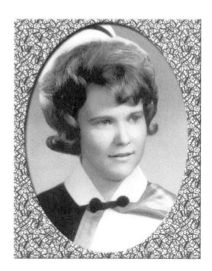

*Judith graduated from St. Joseph's Hospital School of Nursing, Glace Bay, in 1965. She returned to her rural Cape Breton community of Inverness and enjoyed a long and varied career in a small hospital. Her memories capture the joys and heartaches of knowing most of her patients and the pleasure she received from bedside nursing.*

During training I was so intrigued by everything because I had absolutely nothing to do with hospitals; I was never even inside of one and didn't even know anyone who was ill. All of a sudden I had all of this and it was an awakening. I think the thing that bothered me most was the fact that by my second year I was the only one that was from out of town. We had only one day off a week and I couldn't get home, but there were three particular girls that would take me home with them. There was one mom at Whitney Pier and she said: "as long as you are here, my home is your home and when you have a day off, you hop on that bus and come spend it with me." I remember those things so much.

In my second year, I remember calling home because I was really homesick. My mother asked me if I hated it down there or is there something else I would like to do. I told her: "No, I like it when I was on the floors" and she told me to stick to it. And I loved it, even though I think back today about all the changes and it is difficult now with the long shifts. Even though I might growl, I would do it all over again.

First year, I worked in medical, surgical and cardiac. This covered the first floor as it was a small hospital. Also, the emergency room was on this floor, so if something came up, you had to do emergency. We also had to take calls for the OR, you did everything. I did relief supervising for thirteen years and then it was general duty. Obstetrics was my favorite and this was where I was posted 90 per cent of my career. Least favourite would have to be medical nursing. I was never head nurse, but the position was offered to me. But I enjoyed the bedside nursing. I would help with relief. I was also offered the job of in-service coordinator but I wouldn't take it because I loved bedside nursing.

Sometimes you would have a patient who was in a bad accident, who was not expected to live, but would recover and then walk out of the hospital. This is when you say to yourself: "This is what it's all about." I loved obstetrics and I think early on when you had a baby, you were in the hospital for ten days. All these patients that I had are all my friends now and I could get in my car and drop in on them at anytime. And now you have their kids coming in. I loved that aspect of the small hospital. You could come in one day and be in surgical, then the next day it could be something different.

I had a friend who I helped deliver four of her children and then one day her husband came in, and later died, on my shift. I said I would tell her. Then over the next two consecutive shifts, I lost two more patients and that just tore me apart. I had to go off and have a cry to myself. In a small place you pretty much know everyone.

In the nights you would have to go down to emergency if the emergency buzzer rang and you would hold your breath and think: "Who is coming in the doors?" A lot of times it wasn't just close friends, it could be some of my immediate family and you just pull yourself together.

We had a bad fire here and a grandfather and his daughter died. He died saving his grandson's life and I was on for that. That was the worst. I had known the grandmother for a lot of deliveries and they didn't live too far from me. When the family came in that night you just had to take a deep breath and regroup. We were there until about 10 a.m. Coming home you could smell the smoke on your clothes. At this time we had nobody to talk to and debrief us. I wasn't sleeping well for months. We talked about it and went to the director and told her that if this happens again the nurses will need someone to talk to. I can't even enjoy a campfire anymore because it was so traumatic. I see the little boy now, grown up, and he only has a little scarring from the third degree burns he suffered.

I remember I was at a staff meeting one day and our supervisor was very upset because we got a call from a patient's family. This patient was going in for surgery and everyone seemed to know about it. Before this, I was sitting at the desk and the patient was on the phone calling people and telling them that she was in the hospital and having surgery. In a small hospital this happens a lot of the times. You would get asked lots of questions outside of work. People asking what is wrong with so and so. I would just say: "I wasn't in or I don't know."

I think it is still very important to wear your name bar out of respect. I agree with that, but I never felt the uniform and the cap—especially in the last fifteen years—make the nurse. It was the person that made the nurse. They have to get more nurses and give them more training. As far as the degree program, a lot of people cannot afford it. Another thing is that four years is a long time for the hospitals to wait when they need the nurses so desperately.

I retired because I was ready to go. I had worked 37 years and I had always said that I would know when it was time to go. I was getting older, I was 58, and there was a big change in nursing with a shortage and being overworked. It was getting so busy, I found you couldn't spend the time with the patients. I retired in 2002. I am enjoying my retirement, but I enjoyed every bit of my career.

## GLORIA (MATHESON) LEBLANC

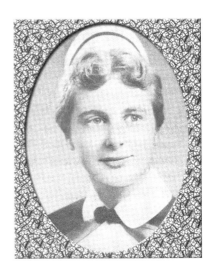

*Gloria graduated from St. Joseph's in 1957. She worked briefly in Cheticamp and moved to Montreal where she nursed for twelve years. Gloria returned to Cheticamp in the early 1970s and worked for twenty-five years, retiring as Director of Nursing in 1996. She remains active in her community as a municipal councillor. She has fond memories of her career in the big city and in her small hospital in Cheticamp.*

When I graduated from high school I was sixteen, so I was too young to go into training. At that time they allowed you to teach school with what they called a permissive licence. It was a very interesting experience. It was a little country school, grade primary to grade eight, forty kids. I knew it wasn't for me, but I just basically enjoyed being with people.

Coming from the country, Glace Bay was a big city to me and I was really scared. I think that at seventeen or eighteen years old, sometimes your thinking process is not geared to what is right. The nuns did your picking for you, but I think they were good at pointing you in the right direction. The three-year training that we got was a lot of hard work and studying and you learned to discipline yourself. You knew that if you went out and didn't get back in at ten o'clock and get to bed early that when the morning bell rang at 5:45 and you didn't get up bright eyed and bushy tailed, you had problems. The first six months you were in the classroom. Then you worked as a "probie" on the floor and the studying came second—but you made sure you got it done. With the nuns, this was their way of life; if you made a mistake, you paid for it. You were grounded like a little kid, you were not allowed out for two weeks. You pulled extra duty, they got their point across. You protected one another and you helped one another. If you got into trouble, you knew someone had your back.

When I graduated in 1957, I spent a year and a half in Cheticamp. I was in surgery, a scrub nurse in the OR. Then I went to Montreal. That was a reality shock. You walk into a hospital like the Jewish General or the Royal Victoria and look up and ask: "What am I doing here?" I spent a total of three years wondering where I was. You are running around trying to orient yourself. The last seven of twelve years I worked at the Jewish Convalescent and Rehab Centre. Patients with heart conditions, accident victims that needed physio—that I really enjoyed. I worked a lot with seniors in Montreal. They can enrich your life for sure. When I worked at the rehab centre you had people who had accidents. It is very rewarding when you have someone who has had surgery or had a major accident and you see him or her back on their feet, ready to go home again. That is what it is all about. It was a time when they had these new medications for Parkinson's Disease. There were ten patients they were doing these medication trials on. It started during the time that I was there. The reason we left and came back was that the political situation was scary and dangerous at that time with the FLQ (Front de liberation du Québec) crisis.

We came back and settled in Cheticamp and I worked for another twenty-five years. The hospital had thirty-nine beds, it had maternity, surgery and all the different departments, serving all the local communities. During my last years, I was Director of Nursing. We started our own version of a home care program. I tried to teach the nurses, especially the younger grads, to be pleasant; be polite but stand up for yourself. If you are right and you feel you are being preyed upon by someone, defend yourself and I will stand behind you. Nursing is hard work and emotionally it is a difficult job. One of the most difficult things to me was coping with people dying, especially accidents.

Most people that come into the hospital don't trust the health care system so you have to gain that trust. Your conversational skills have to be good. In a small country hospital where everybody knows everybody else, one of the things that really has to be impressed upon nurses is that one single word can give things away about a patient and hit the gossip mills. Basically, country folks, we do that, not because it is gossip, but because we care.

To me, nursing was my life. I graduated, I went to work, I married and I had a family and worked all the way through. In my day, there was no such thing as maternity leave or unemployment. I had my children and went back to work.

Hopefully we are going to go back to some sort of program that would provide enough nurses because I am getting to an age that one of these days I might end up in a hospital or a nursing home and I want to see nurses around. What is happening right now is that nurses are getting really scarce and are overworked, getting burnt out and it is not good for health care. So I am hoping that there will be some happy medium, whether it be a two- or three-year program so that we will have more nurses in order to provide decent health care.

## HEATHER LeBLANC

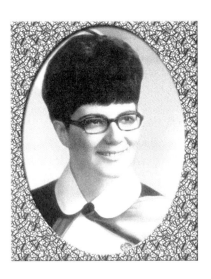

*Heather graduated from St. Rita in 1969 and worked in Newfoundland for a year before returning to Cape Breton and beginning a 33-year career at the small community hospital in Cheticamp. She worked on surgical units, in the OR and outpatients and in administration. Heather retired in 2003. She reflects on the joys of nursing in a small community and the challenges of managing care in a cash-strapped system.*

I went into training in 1966 and graduated in 1969. We were like a happy family and we lived in residence. I lived in Sydney; in fact I lived right across from the hospital, but in those days they wanted you to live in residence. Some days you didn't think it was all that great, but when you look back you know it was good. My mother was housemother at the residence. It was nice to have her there. She was tougher on me because she couldn't show favouritism. We had a lot of on the job training which was good at the time. We would be in class in the morning and have to go on the floors in afternoon to work. We did a lot of work and you didn't dare say anything, you just did it. Some days you felt you were just there cleaning, but I suppose we were learning discipline. We spent a lot of time talking to the patients and I know they enjoyed having the students around.

First year we were probies, on probation. We would go on the floor. If you passed all of your exams you got a cap and a uniform and that summer you worked on the floor. In September, you got a yellow band and a stipend of $8 a month. Of course that went a little further than it does now. It went up to $10 the following spring. We would get a blue band and then it went up to $12. We worked the summers and at Christmas. You would get three weeks off in the summer. It wasn't like university today, not at all. During the summer the staff would have vacation and you were there. It was good experience. During the last year, you were given a chance to be in charge of the floor. It was scary but exciting and you knew what nursing was all about.

I went to Newfoundland because when I came out of nursing there were no jobs at St. Rita. In fact there were no jobs in Nova Scotia. There was an abundance of nurses that year. Things changed after that. I went to Newfoundland, to Corner Brook. They were desperately short of nurses. So the first day I walked in there, of course I was going to change everything. They put me in a room to "special" these two patients that were both in accidents the night before. There was no ICU, they were specialed in their room and I found out that I was not going to change things. I stayed in Newfoundland for a year and then came to Cheticamp for three months. Well, it was supposed to be three months. I was supposed to go to the Halifax Infirmary. I stayed in Cheticamp and was there for thirty-three years. I met my husband and we got married and had a daughter.

I started in Cheticamp as a staff nurse. I was on the surgical unit on the first floor. I started in 1970 and my daughter was born in 1974. At that time we were allowed six weeks before and six weeks after so I worked until about two weeks before I was due. I took the other weeks when I had her. When those six weeks were up, they were really desperate. I went back to work and thought nothing of it. I had a babysitter and when you live in a small community, my husband's sister lived just up the road, so she took over. Then I started working in the OR and we had surgery two days a week so on those two days I'd be in the OR and the other days I was on the floor. Then I took over in charge of the OR and outpatients as well and I really loved that. I did that until 1994 and then I took over as Director of Patient Care/Nursing.

I have done my nursing administrative program through a university in Ontario. I have done a chemotherapy course and that was part of my job the last five years. That is very rewarding because you are helping people. The patient does not have to go to Sydney. That was a big success being part of that. One of the difficulties is your budget, there is never enough money, as Director of Nursing I was seeing that. We had a few bad years when cutbacks were made and people that were left behind felt they were doing the job of two people.

I retired in 2003 because I was the magic age and I felt it was time to pass it on to a younger person. I never thought I would like geriatrics, but since I retired, I was going to go and volunteer to feed patients and the administrator of the nursing home said: "We are looking for a nurse; instead of volunteering, come and work for a day." They are so happy to see you and so appreciative, completely different than a hospital.

## MARY (CHISHOLM) FLECK

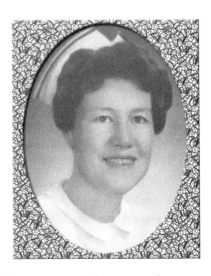

*Mary began her nursing career as a nurse's aid in the United States in 1965. She later trained as a licenced practical nurse and finally as an RN, graduating from Mount Wachusett Nursing School in Gardner, Massachusetts, in 1976. This mother of nine children began her career in obstetrics in Massachusetts. In 1978, she moved to Cape Breton and began working at the Inverness Consolidated Hospital. Mary retired in 1991.*

I am not really sure why I wanted to be a nurse. I do remember that my next-door neighbour, when I was very small, was a student nurse and when she came home and did her laundry there were those beautiful black stockings she hung on the clothes line.

I entered the nursing field as a nurse's aid in 1965, being married and having eight children. In 1968, I entered an LPN program at a state hospital for the mentally ill. This, for me, was the very worst of my entire nursing experience. Many of these patients had been used to test the newly-introduced tranquilizers and were suffering the long term effects. Many had been in for thirty or forty years, abandoned by families and with no home to go to.

There were a few male nurses. They were not well treated, mostly used for lifting or managing difficult, disoriented patients. Their nursing education was hardly ever used. By the time I had completed my nursing education, there were many more males and they were treated as nurses.

In 1972, I entered Mount Wachusett Community College in Gardner, Massachusetts, and graduated in 1976 with an Associate of Science in Nursing. By now I had nine children and am proud that I graduated with honours. I was very proud, not only of me, but my family. My husband, who had been so supportive in it, helped with housework and cooking and child care, and of my children who were just about as helpful. The nicest thing when I graduated was hearing from people whom I had attended as a student. They sent cards, called me and even stopped me on the street to congratulate me and tell me some little story.

Immediately after getting my RN, I worked on the obstetrics floor. My greatest memory was the first time I saw a baby born, the thrill of a new life. Another is the first time I saw a successful resuscitation. Throughout my career, I worked in pediatrics. It was okay, but not as great as obstetrics. Pre- and post-op, I liked this. ICU: very challenging, always had to be on your toes. It could be exhausting, but I like it. And step-down: I didn't care to work there. My favourite was obstetrics. Although there were some sad incidents, it was mostly a very pleasant place to work.

Lifelong friendships were made during training and working. A joy was the wonderful reception I had as a stranger from most of the nurses in Inverness when I arrived from the States to work here. The help they gave me in some techniques and names of some medications that differed from those I was used to. The laughs we had when someone used a Caper expression I was unfamiliar with. Or at my Boston accent.

Depending upon the patient, I have felt like I was a teacher explaining what and why; a child performing a task in the way an elderly patient wanted it done; a clergyman with a dying patient wanting to pray or have his bible read; a friend for the patient whose family was not around or may have abandoned him; a housekeeper trying to keep a clean area for an unsteady or incompetent patient; mother or grandmother for a frightened child.

I retired early in 1991. The decision came on a stormy January night travelling to work in Inverness. On this twenty-mile trip, I met one snowplow coming in the opposite direction and not one car. It took me well over an hour to make that trip on and off the road and lots of prayers. Since I worked nearly all nights as a supervisor, I felt I had had enough. The next day I submitted my resignation after thirteen years.

I don't think I like the idea of nurses not wearing caps or uniforms. I feel that the patients feel less security about their care when they are not sure who is doing their care. I have been told this a few times by people who have been hospitalized. The doctor/nurse relationship has improved; the nurse is considered more of a partner in patient care, but I see the distance between the nurse and patient becoming much greater. The RN's role is becoming more of a desk job, more papers to fill in, more teaching of other patient care personnel. I see less and less bonding between the RN and patient. That is too bad.

1977: The new 75-bed Inverness Consolidated Hospital opened in Inverness, replacing two smaller facilities and serving 9,000 residents in a 50-mile radius.

# RICHMOND COUNTY

> 1946: The Canadian Red Cross established a hospital in Arichat.

## MARGARET (MARCHAND) CUSACK

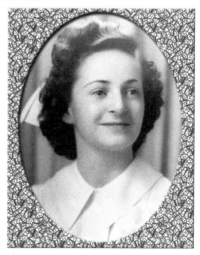

*Margaret graduated from St. Joseph's Hospital School of Nursing, Glace Bay, in 1944 and began work on a surgical floor at the Halifax Infirmary during the war years. After three years, she nursed for a summer on a Montreal neurological unit and returned to Cape Breton as Matron of a Red Cross Hospital in Arichat. Margaret left her career in 1949 to raise a family of eight children. She went back to work briefly in the 1960s. Margaret recalls the mid-century medical advances she witnessed and compares her work with the modern nursing role.*

I guess I decided to become a nurse because of the influence of a friend of my parents who had trained at St. Joseph's and thought I should go there. That was one of the reasons. I had taught school for a year with a permissive licence. I entered training in 1941. I loved being in residence and the association with all the girls. We didn't really love the ten o'clock curfew that we had. We went through the three years with just two weeks vacation and it was a seven-days-a-week thing. If we were on night duty for instance, we had classes in the afternoon. We went to bed in the morning and got up in the afternoon to go to classes.

It was during the war years and nurses were very scarce at that time, so I went from Glace Bay to the Halifax Infirmary. I was on the surgical floor and I liked that very much. It was a shock because it was a lot bigger [than Glace Bay]. The Sisters of St. Martha ran the hospital in Glace Bay and the Infirmary was run by the Sisters of Charity. They had different rules than we were accustomed to. I worked there for three years. After that I went to Montreal and worked at the neurological for a summer. I would have stayed there, I loved it there, but I got a call to come home to Arichat. They had opened an outpost Red Cross hospital and they wanted me to be the matron. It sounded like a very wonderful job but, as it turned out I was not only the matron, but the full-time nurse. I had to order all the supplies and look after the whole administration on a salary of $80 a month for a 12, 16, sometimes 24-hour day.

The Red Cross Hospital served an area that had not previously had access to hospital facilities ... those of us on staff felt we were filling a real need. We had experiences of serving people that would probably have died without the hospital in their community. I recall a patient, a farmer, admitted to the hospital. He was thought to have arthritis. He went into a spasm. We called the doctor and after consultation with the Department of Health, the patient was diagnosed with tetanus. The doctor used a low dosage of Sodium Pentothal to bring him out of the spasm. The doctor said to me: "when he goes into spasms like this and I am out on call, we might lose him. I will show you how to administer it and you have to be very careful with it." Sure enough, I had to give it him. It was scary, but those were the things we had to do in a crisis situation. The patient lived to go back to his farm.

We were on a very strict budget. We had very little money. That is why Medicare is so important. You have no idea the difference in today compared to when we nursed. The biggest change I had seen was when penicillin came in, probably the last year of our training. It was such a wonderful drug, a miracle drug, it really was.

I think a little bit of you dies with every patient, especially when they are young or children.

Male nurses were discriminated against. Some people felt it really wasn't a job for a man and they were not given as much credit as they should have been. For instance, they were not allowed in the case room and did mostly male catheterization and that type of thing.

I loved nursing and I was sorry to leave when I had my family. I retired, I guess, in 1949. I did go back and take a refresher course and thought I would go back into nursing, but I had eight kids so I had a little bit of responsibility at home. I could not handle both so I stayed home. I went back to nursing, probably in the late 60s for about two years on and off.

I would not want to be nursing today, the kind of nursing we did was bedside nursing. I admire what the nurses today can do, but I would not want to do all the paperwork. It is a very difficult profession. I have been a patient recently and nurses are still doing some bedside nursing and they are every bit as good at it as we think we were.

> 1962: Residents of the Canso Strait area called for a new hospital.

## VI (MANCINI) SAMPSON

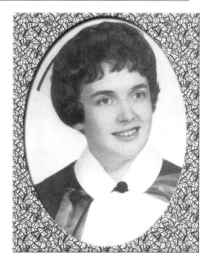

*Vi graduated from St. Elizabeth's Hospital, North Sydney, in 1962 and began her career at St. Martha's Hospital in Antigonish. She returned to Cape Breton a year later, married and started a family. Vi returned to nursing in the 1970s and worked for thirty years in a St. Peter's nursing home. She retired as Director of Nursing in 2003. Her love of gerontology is evident in her career memories.*

I wanted to follow in my sister's footsteps. When I was younger, playing with my dolls, they were always sick in bed or bandaged with a sheet.

We were a close knit class, the class of '62. It was just a bonding. The highlight of my training days was meeting them because being from a country area, I was very shy. I had some senior nurses that took me under their wing. The first six months was hard because I wanted to go home. I had a sister who lived in North Sydney who was a nurse and that helped me, too. I felt it was very overwhelming. It was a lot to absorb just coming out of high school. If I had to do it over again today, I would have waited a year or two.

After graduation, I felt prepared and I wanted to explore a different setting. I could probably have worked in the hospital where I trained, but I chose to go to Antigonish to St. Martha's for a year, which I enjoyed very much. I worked in third west, which was post-op. I worked there from November to October of the following year and, in October, I went to the small hospital in Arichat. I got married in June. When I had my children, I did not work from 1965 to 1969. In 1969 when MSI came into effect, I worked in St. Peter's for a local doctor, just eight hours a week, like a nurse/receptionist. I did that until 1972 and then I went to the nursing home. I was there for thirty years.

The joys in gerontology were the knowledge, the wit and the wisdom of the elderly. That is what keeps you motivated. They have so much to offer and they are so eager for your company. You can do your medication rounds, probably in an hour-and-a-half, but it would take you four hours because they wanted to tell you who was in visiting during the day, or if they had a new great granddaughter or so-and-so is getting married. You would have to stop and listen. The heartache was when you would get attached to someone and they would pass away. You try not to do that but over the years, it is hard not to. We now have palliative care from the local hospital and there are a lot of volunteers. If we have a resident that has no family, they assign a couple, especially if they are acutely ill, to be with them the last couple of weeks. That was a big thing for me, not to have anyone pass away alone. Even if they can sense you are there, they will turn their head toward you. Another heartache is the Alzheimer patients. There is so much agitation and turmoil with those clients ... to see what they go through. The last fifteen years that I was there, you really had to be on top of the new programming, all kinds of courses. We are getting younger clients with MS. They have so much courage. They are very mentally alert and they realize they are suffering. Some people are handed such crosses to bear.

My most memorable accomplishment, I guess, was being able to ladder myself from staff nurse to head nurse to director of care. I was very active in gerontology, I took an extended care management program through the Canadian Hospital Association. I did that in 1976 to be able to apply for more jobs in gerontology. One of the handicaps we had was that we were not appropriately funded for the needs of the first ten or fifteen years I was there. Our rate wasn't covering enough to provide education for the care givers and equipment to look after the elderly and the disabled. In 1996, the Department of Health took us over and the change in the two years following was phenomenal. All our RNs got parity with all others in Nova Scotia. The last five years of working was a dream. We got electric beds, a couple of lifts and a whirlpool bath. We had seventy-five beds in the nursing home. Just before I left, I was on a steering committee to build a new one and it is still ongoing.

I left in 2003, after thirty years, and my husband had been retired for five years. I would like to have worked a couple of more, but there were a lot of issues the last couple of years. I was Director of Nursing and it was just a nightmare, especially in summer. I would not get a good night's sleep because I would worry that someone would call in sick and what would I do to replace them, so the stress factor.... I am just getting used to retirement now. I am on the community health board as a volunteer.

---

1978: Deputy Prime Minister Allan J. MacEachern turned the sod to officially begin construction of the $4 million Strait-Richmond Hospital. The 48-bed hospital, located at Inhabitants River, would employ 100 people.

---

# INDEX

## B

Phyllis Ball  110
Grace (Whalen) Bonnar  74
Lenora Brewster  48
Eleanor (Morrison) Burke  64

## C

Betty Jane Cameron  162
Roberta (MacMillan) Cameron  157
Lynne (Walker) Clarke  88
Ethel (Squarey) Cluett  135
Geraldeen (Butler) Collins  41
Betty Cordeau (Elizabeth)  85
Anita (Skinner) Cousins  44
Jock Crosby 40
Jessie (Kavanaugh) Curtis  143
Margaret (Marchand) Cusack  177

## D

Ann (Campbell) D'Andrea  101
Alfreda Douglas  137
Betty (MacLellan) Dowe  51

## F

Janice Ferguson  165
Mary (Chisholm) Fleck  174
Marilyn Morrison Foley  120
Alice (MacLean) Freeman  159
Irene (Stephenson) Funge  116

## G

Judith (Ferguson) Gillis  167
Tula (Mancini) Gouthro  123
Thelma (Timmons) Grant  139

## H

Jean (MacInnis) Hemsworth  35
Marion (MacLean) Hopkins  46

## J

Jane (DeLeskie) Jessome  132
Amelia (Sylliboy) Jesty  127

## L

Gloria (Matheson) LeBlanc  170
Heather LeBlanc  172

## M

Emma (MacLean) MacDonald  58
Marion (Mitchell) MacDonald  77

Norma (MacKinnon) MacDonald  28
Shirley MacDonald  100
Edna (Farquhar) MacDougall  82
Dr. Marion (Atkinson) MacIntosh  95
Christina (MacDonald) MacIntyre  26
Mary (Cleary) MacIssac  122
Laura (Watts) MacKinnon  67
Emily (MacLean) MacLeod  147
Irene (Herve) MacMillan  62
Hannah (MacDonald) Matheson  145
Sister Veronica Matthews  106
Frances (Doucette) McIntyre  104
Mary Lee (Waters) Morrison  160
Sister Barbara Muldoon  60

## O

Effie (MacDougall) Ormiston  30
Albert Orrell  80

## P

Caroline (Gromick) Paruch  93
Elsie (Dakai) Percy  79
Judy (Burden) Price  53

## R

Carole Ravanello  108
Dr. Simone Roach  32
Ann (Goss) Robinson  125

## S

Vi (Mancini) Sampson  179
Gladys (Philips) Smith  37
Rita (Jones) Smith  155
Ann Marie (Day) (Grandy) Steele  130
Kathleen Stephenson  118
Jim Struthers  98

## T

Claire (Roach) Timmons  69

## W

Tina (Matthews) Waters  160
Natalie Wilkie 113
Regina (Donovan) Williams  152
Sharon (Donovan) Williams  150

## Y

Clotilda (Coward) (Douglas) Yakimchuk  90

Sincere thanks to the many people and organizations who made the project possible.

Dr. Raed Azer
Cape Breton Council of Seniors and Pensioners
Cara Leah Hmidan
Carefield Manor Ltd.
CAW Local 198 Dairy Workers
Cape Breton Economic Development Authority
Cape Breton Regional Municipality
Dr. Joseph Claener
Community Employment Innovation Project (CEIP)
Kim Conrad (in memory of mother)
Betty Cordeau (in memory of her family)
Dr. P Creighton
Cusack Law Office Inc.
Glace Bay Local N.S.N.U./CBRH
Francis Healy
Hip-Hip-Hooray – Dr. Kevin Orrell
Dr. C. Hobbs
Human Resources and Social Development Canada
Dr. Yolanda D'Intino
Joneljim Concrete Construction
Iwanis Ceilidh Golden K
Dr. Mandat Maharaj
Maple Hill Manor
Merck Frost Canada
Mr. Arnie Mombourquette (in memory of mother who was a nurse)
New Waterford Local N.S.N./CBRH
Otarion Hearing Aid Centre Ltd.
Dr. M. N. Patel
Pharmasave Drug Store
Province of Nova Scotia Office of Economic Development
Ratchford Photographic Studio
Dr. J. A. Roach
Roche Pharmaceutical Ltd.
Rudderham Chernin Law Office Inc.
Shannex Health Group
Dr. Murdock Smith
Sobey's Prince Street
Steele City Credit Union

Kathleen/Irene Stephenson/Funge
(in memory of mother and father)
Steve Lewis Auto Body
Sydney Credit Union
Sydney Local N.S.U./CBRH
Sydney Memorial Chapel
Sydney Steelworkers Pensioner's Club
T. W. Curry Parkview Chapel
Whitney Credit Union Ltd.

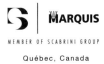

MEMBER OF SCABRINI GROUP

Québec, Canada
2007